Food and Public Health

T0227604

This book focuses on food policy, and its relationship to public health, as an increasingly important issue in today's society. Contributors highlight the lack of global regulation in the food supply chain and explore the common tendency to leave regulation to markets and to individual consumer decisions. In a period where there is growing concern about the sustainability of contemporary food systems, this book considers the inadequate response made to issues of food waste where solutions in high income countries are dependent on lifestyle and consumer behaviour. It offers an insight in to the importance of people's everyday lives in relation to policies on public health, food and sustainability. The text demonstrates the corrosive impact of social inequality, and the futility of identifying lower income consumers as flawed when aiming for food policies that seek to achieve improvements in public health. Factors such as technological developments, ecological concerns and international trade are also taken in to account.

This book was originally published as a special issue of *Critical Public Health*.

Dr Wendy Wills is a Reader in Food and Public Health in the Centre for Research in Primary and Community Care (CRIPACC) at the University of Hertfordshire, UK. She is a Sociologist and Nutritionist (Public Health).

Dr Alizon Draper is a Reader in Public Health Nutrition at the University of Westminster, UK. She has a background in social anthropology and her work has focused on the social and policy aspects of nutrition.

Ulla Gustafsson is a Principal Lecturer at the University of Roehampton, UK. She is a Medical Sociologist with interests in food policy and public health.

Food and Public Health
Contemporary Issues and Future Directions

Edited by
**Wendy Wills, Alizon Draper and
Ulla Gustafsson**

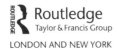 Routledge
Taylor & Francis Group

LONDON AND NEW YORK

First published 2013
by Routledge
2 Park Square, Milton Park, Abingdon, Oxfordshire OX14 4RN

Simultaneously published in the USA and Canada
by Routledge
711 Third Avenue, New York, NY 10017

First issued in paperback 2015

Routledge is an imprint of the Taylor & Francis Group, an informa business

© 2013 Taylor & Francis

This book is a reproduction of *Critical Public Health*, Volume 21, Issue 4. The Publisher requests to those authors who may be citing this book to state, also, the bibliographical details of the special issue on which the book was based.

All rights reserved. No part of this book may be reprinted or reproduced or utilised in any form or by any electronic, mechanical, or other means, now known or hereafter invented, including photocopying and recording, or in any information storage or retrieval system, without permission in writing from the publishers.

Trademark notice: Product or corporate names may be trademarks or registered trademarks, and are used only for identification and explanation without intent to infringe.

British Library Cataloguing in Publication Data
A catalogue record for this book is available from the British Library

ISBN13: 978-1-138-94393-3 (pbk)
ISBN13: 978-0-415-65962-8 (hbk)

Typeset in Times New Roman
by Taylor & Francis Books

Publisher's Note
The publisher would like to make readers aware that the chapters in this book may be referred to as articles as they are identical to the articles published in the special issue. The publisher accepts responsibility for any inconsistencies that may have arisen in the course of preparing this volume for print.

Contents

CONTENTS

Citation Information

The following chapters were originally published in the journal *Critical Public Health.* When citing this material, please use the original issue information and page numbering for each article, as follows:

Chapter 7

Blaming the consumer – once again: the social and material contexts of everyday food waste practices in some English households
David Evans
Critical Public Health, volume 21, issue 4 (December 2011) pp. 429-440

Chapter 8

Health improvement, nutrition-related behaviour and the role of school meals: the usefulness of a socio-ecological perspective to inform policy design, implementation and evaluation
Sue N. Moore, Simon Murphy and Laurence Moore
Critical Public Health, volume 21, issue 4 (December 2011) pp. 441-454

Chapter 9

Food insecurity in South Australian single parents: an assessment of the livelihoods framework approach
Iain R. Law, Paul R. Ward and John Coveney
Critical Public Health, volume 21, issue 4 (December 2011) pp. 455-469

Chapter 10

Doing 'healthier' food in everyday life? A qualitative study of how Pakistani Danes handle nutritional communication
Bente Halkier and Iben Jensen
Critical Public Health, volume 21, issue 4 (December 2011) pp. 471-483

Chapter 11

A focus group study of food safety practices in relation to listeriosis among the over-60s
Richard Milne
Critical Public Health, volume 21, issue 4 (December 2011) pp. 485-495

Chapter 12

Preventing anxiety: a qualitative study of fish consumption and pregnancy
Helene Brembeck
Critical Public Health, volume 21, issue 4 (December 2011) pp. 497-508

Notes on Contributors

Helene Brembeck, University of Gothenburg, Sweden

Claudia Chaufan, University of California San Francisco, USA

Rosemary Collier, University of Warwick, UK

Sophia Constantino, University of California San Francisco, USA

John Coveney, Flinders University, Australia

Meagan Davis, University of California San Francisco, USA

Roberto De Vogli, University of Michigan, USA and University College London, UK

Elizabeth A. Dowler, University of Warwick, UK

Alizon Draper, University of Westminster, London, UK

David Evans, University of Manchester, UK

Patrick Fox, University of California San Francisco, USA

David Gimeno, The University of Texas Health Science Center at Houston, USA

Ulla Gustafsson, Roehampton University, London, UK

Bente Halkier, Roskilde University, Denmark

Gee Hee Hong, University of California San Francisco, USA

Andreas Hirseland, Institut für Arbeitsmarkt- und Berufsforschung, Germany

Alex Inman, Alex Inman Consulting, UK

Iben Jensen, Roskilde University, Denmark

Moya Kneafsey, Coventry University, UK

Anne Kouvonen, Warsaw School of Social Sciences and Humanities, Wroclaw Faculty, Wroclaw, Poland

Hannah Lambie, Applied Research Centre in Sustainable Regeneration, Futures Institute, UK

Iain R. Law, Flinders University, Australia

Richard Milne, University of Sheffield, UK

Laurence Moore, Cardiff University, UK

Sue N. Moore, Cardiff University, UK

Simon Murphy, Cardiff University, UK

Sabine Pfeiffer, Institut für Sozialwissenschaftliche Forschung e.V. München, Germany

Tobias Ritter, Institut für Sozialwissenschaftliche Forschung e.V. München, Germany

Paul R. Ward, Flinders University, Australia

Wendy Wills, CRIPACC, University of Hertfordshire, UK

Food and public health: contemporary issues and future directions

Ulla Gustafsson
Department of Social Sciences, Roehampton University, London, UK

Wendy Wills
CRIPACC, University of Hertfordshire, UK

Alizon Draper
School of Life Sciences, University of Westminster, London, UK

The British Sociological Association's Food Study Group held their second international conference on *Food, Society and Public Health* in 2010, and a selection of papers presented at this event is included in this volume, along with other, complementary, papers published in Critical Public Health. A key focus for debate centred on food security and sustainability, an area of considerable import for public health.

In 2003, *Critical Public Health* published a Special Issue on food that stressed the importance of food policy for public health (Coveney 2003). Urging a *politics of food* perspective, Coveney identified an inherent policy tension between the promotion of health and facilitating trade in ensuring the food supply; such tension points to the potential for conflict in regulation. In the same year, Caraher and Coveney (2003, p. 591) took issue with the narrow focus in public health nutrition on 'dietary guidelines and lifestyle factors'. They urged an 'upstream' approach to food policy in order to address the negative impact on the environment and public health from the current shape of the global food market. Nearly a decade later, the issue of regulation remains problematic and clashes of interests abound. For example, Thornley et al. (2010) show how the New Zealand advertising standards system is failing to hold the self-regulated industry to account when it comes to upholding the rights of children. Similarly, consumer failure depicted as the result of consumers making poor choices rather than a critique of the quality in the supply chain is still the focus when considering poor diets (Harris et al. 2009). Further, income inequalities are growing ever wider and there are increasing signs of food poverty, even in high-income countries, adding to the number of hungry worldwide (Dowler et al., Pfeiffer et al., this volume). Environmental questions such as biodiversity, the contribution of agriculture to climate change and degradation of land were also topical at the time, with Coveney (2003) and Caraher and Coveney (2003) identifying concerns that remain on the contemporary policy agenda. However, food security and sustainability have become all the more prominent.

The focus on food security and sustainability has led to a greater sense of urgency for immediate action. A number of recent reports have highlighted the need to ensure a sustainable food system in order to avoid irreversible damage (DFID 2010, Food Ethics Council 2010, Foresight 2011, Oxfam 2011). This is partly due to the challenge posed by recent volatility in the food system (Foresight 2011). In 2008, there were riots in countries across the world as a result of the dramatic increase in the cost of food that was caused by a number of contributing factors to do with climate change, lack of regulation and market fluctuations (Foresight 2011). The number of people who went hungry peaked at over one billion in 2008. This signalled a new precariousness with regard to food prices that in the previous 20-year period had remained fairly stable by comparison. Continued warnings about rises in prices for maize by 105% and wheat by 102% between March 2010 and March 2011 have serious implications for the one billion who live on $1 per day (von Braun 2011). While the Millennium goals to reduce hunger look unattainable, we are made acutely aware that the poorest in our world are extremely vulnerable. A third of children in developing countries remain undernourished, with serious implications for healthy development (DFID 2010).

In addition to instability in food prices, we have been reminded of the potentially destructive effects of climate change through a number of recent devastating natural disasters, alerting us to the need to plan for uncertainty. Sustainability has particular salience therefore as the effects of climate change are seen as posing a particular challenge to the food system. Foresight (2011) identifies a number of priorities for action, including the reduction of waste. Here it is noted that in high-income countries waste is more a problem at the consumer end, while it is located at the producer end in low-income countries. Reduction of waste is considered 'an area where individual citizens and businesses . . . can make a clear contribution' (p. 36). Waste disposal is framed as a consumer choice and yet another feature of contemporary life that citizens have to engage with. It is an example of the trend towards a reduction in state involvement prevalent in contemporary society. Parfitt et al. (2010, p. 3079) argue that 'changes in legislation and business behaviour towards more sustainable food production' is necessary as they do not hold much hope that changes in consumer behaviour will be effective. Current policy continues to pass the safeguarding of health onto the individual despite evidence of its inadequacy. Sustainability is a further area now devolved to individual responsibility with the promotion of so-called pro-environmental behaviours. As such it is illustrative of current forms of neo-liberal governance. 'The modern subject has responsibilities not just towards the self, but to the political body, as a new kind of citizenship emerges, with its emphasis on engagement and empowerment' (Green and Labonté 2008, p. 9). In the most recent UK Government policy on public health in England, people are to be 'nudged' into adopting healthier life styles (Department of Health 2010). This signals a rejection of direct state intervention and reliance instead on public engagement at the individual level.

Food security and sustainability are high up on the agenda of many governments around the world and the Foresight Report (2011) offers considered proposals for policy makers in advocating a focus on the global food system. Food security and sustainability are necessarily located in global high-level policy formulations and this invariably presents difficulties. Even though there are global level regulations, for example the WTO, there is a distinction in power where economic power is located at a global level while political power remains national (Labonté et al. 2008, p. 16). Such circumstances present different levels of tension. However, when operating at global-level policy, it is often easy to forget the significance of food in sustaining not only the continuity of the world population and its physical health, but also cultural values and social relations. Poland and Dooris (2010) raise some concerns regarding the link between sustainability and health. They note 'that work on sustainability and health have largely been developed in parallel rather than in an integrated manner' (2010, p. 281). In examining the definition of food security adopted at the 1996 World Food Summit, Pottier (1999, p. 11) discusses the difficulties with the discrepancy between 'high-level policy formulations of food security' and 'the complex real-life experiences and perceptions of the food-insecure'. He argues that the solutions offered are often global and technical in nature, are based on poorly defined concepts and take inadequate account of the life of the food insecure. Through ethnographic exploration of perceptions and practices related to food, he identifies a number of difficulties in bridging the gap between global policies ensuring appropriate access to food and how food is actually accessed on the ground.

Pottier's exploration of African ethnographies illustrates the significance of food in social and cultural life. This is evident in the sociology of food that has emerged over the last few decades that point to the extensive meanings attached to food also in high-income countries (Wills 2011). However, in contemporary public health discourse, health tends to predominate while social and cultural discourses are downplayed. Lindsay (2010, p. 475) argues that there is a 'disconnect' between healthy eating guidelines, that assume an 'idealised, individualised world', and actual practices in everyday life. In this context, it is relevant to consider de Certeau's (1984) work on everyday life. His work is a reaction to Foucault's concept of 'disciplinary society' which de Certeau felt neglected to explain how an entire society can resist the expansion of 'discipline'. De Certeau (1984) argues that it is important to study everyday life in its own right and it is in the routines of everyday, mundane practices that we can detect ways in which power is resisted and contested. It is not in grand political gestures that we can detect such resistance but in minor rule breaking in everyday lives. This he refers to as 'making do' (1984, p. 29). It requires us to be able 'to combine heterogeneous elements (thus in the supermarket, the housewife confronts heterogeneous and mobile data – what she has in the refrigerator, the tastes, appetites, and moods of her guests, the best buys and their possible combinations with what she already has on hand at home, etc.); the intellectual synthesis of these given elements takes the form, however, not of a discourse, but of the decision itself, the act and manner in which the opportunity is 'seized' (de Certeau 1984, p. xix).

This example serves as an illustration of the way that a careful study of the everyday can throw light on acts of minor rule breaking such as selecting food for the pleasure it will bring rather than its health effects. It also underlines the complex consideration that public health policies need to engage with when it concerns food. Indeed, Devisch and Dierckz (2009) suggest that a public health policy that considers human desire is likely to include a more realistic premise. The consumerist approach evident in the majority of such policies is often rather narrow and simplistic by comparison.

In examining the ordinary at a micro level, it is nevertheless important to retain a perspective of structural factors as consumer choice is often made in circumstances beyond individual control. Such choice is often shaped by social inequalities in terms of access to healthy food and vulnerability to poor diets and food poisoning. Consequently, Tansey and Rajotte (2008) stress the need to study up- as well as down-stream when exploring (lack of) access to food. Further, van Rijnsoever et al. (2011) argue that consumers desire food for many reasons other than health while producers are ready to meet such demand in view of the profitability associated with the supply of unhealthy products. Van Rijnsoever et al. describe this relationship between consumers and food producers as a 'lock-in' that is impossible to leave to markets alone and that would require policy intervention. The report by the WHO Commission on Social Determinants of Health on health equity makes a number of recommendations that acknowledge structural factors with a view to improve conditions for daily living (CSDH 2008). Indeed, it points to the importance of nutrition in early life and sees food security as crucial in order to ensure this. However, Green (2010) notes there is an emphasis on mid- to down-stream factors rather than a radical action to redistribute power. Bauman's (2011) conceptualisation of inequalities reminds us of the limitations imposed upon well-intentioned and considered global proposals. He points out that inequality is viewed as a financial problem rather than a problem affecting society as a whole. He considers this a corrosive position but one that politicians are drawn to in a neo-liberal world. He employs the military metaphor of 'collateral damage' to explain how the underclass is considered to be outside of normal society and not counting as part of it. Similarly, poverty becomes re-classified as a problem of 'law and order' rather than being seen as a structural feature of society. As a result, people become 'collateral casualty of profit-driven, uncoordinated and uncontrolled globalization' (Bauman 2011, p. 4): the greater the social inequality the larger the number of 'collateral casualties'. What an examination of the everyday contributes in this context is a reminder that even 'collateral casualties' exist in a cultural and social context and that it is important, if the enhancement of public health is the aim, to understand how their structural context contributes to forms of resistance.

This Special Issue reminds us that we need to keep a focus on all aspects of food in public health. As the focus in policy firmly shifts onto food security and sustainability, it can become easy to forget about the crucial part that food serves in everyday life and its role for maintaining physical, social and emotional health. It also serves to repeat the critical account of consumerism and levels of inequality noted in the 2003 Special Issue. We will examine some of the unifying themes in the papers included in this collection followed by outlines of each contribution.

It is in the daily consumption of food that the rationale for food security and sustainability is realised. While food policy is a complex enterprise with multiple connections and interests, it is therefore important to be mindful of the everyday and the way this is affected by and impacts on the policy process. The papers in this collection include reference to the implications of food policy and public health at this level even though none of the studies have explicitly drawn on de Certeau for analysis. Evans' findings demonstrate that food waste is often an act that reflects the way an 'opportunity is "seized"' (de Certeau 1984, p. xix) and as such it is problematic to adopt a simplistic 'rational choice' consumer concept at the policy level. Further, Brembeck's work reveals the potential disruption inflicted on well-informed consumers by the fear of having eaten Baltic herring. Similarly, everyday practices are at the forefront in the way Pakistani Danes may prefer to prepare food for the pleasure it provides rather than its healthiness (Halkier and Jensen). Even when they share the goal of health with health educators, the cultural and social relevance of food cannot be neglected. In Chaufan et al's study of Latinos living in the USA, the burden of being poor and coping with this on a daily basis represented a major barrier to eating a diet conducive to preventing the onset of diabetes. Vulnerability to food poisoning among people over 60 years in England is the topic of Milne's study. While focusing on the food associated social practices among this generation, we see the way that disruption to these practices increases their risk to succumb to food poisoning. Moore's study indicates that top down healthy public policy may be resisted due to the ordinary working practices of staff in primary school dining halls. Finally, Chaufan, Fox and Hong argue that a move towards labelling food outlet menus with calorie information could result in greater, not fewer inequalities in diet and health.

It is important to bear such a perspective in mind when exploring global issues such as food security and sustainability. Food security is a term that has been more commonly applied to low-income countries. Dowler's study shows the relevance of the concept of food security in high-income countries like the UK, where consumers are concerned about the evident increase in food prices. Adults in some households with children reported going without food in order to ensure their children had enough. Furthermore, some respondents acknowledged having to compromise on the quality and healthiness of food due to the cost thus suggesting limits to existing regulation. Chaufan et al's study illustrates similar compromises being made in poor immigrant households in the US and Pfeiffer et al. suggest that the expansion of food banks in Germany signals increasing levels of hunger and food insecurity. Focusing on obesity as a pressing public health problem among the poor provides a way to avoid addressing issues of food security in this high-income country. Australia is another country not associated with hunger although certain groups are found to be more vulnerable than others (Law et al.). Australian single parents reported difficulties in finding true supermarket bargains and also identified the limited range of foods that tend to be included in special offers. The lack of regulation in food policy therefore does little to limit the unequal nutritional vulnerability they face. The implications of inadequate regulations for nutritional, if not food, security is evident in de Vogli et al.'s contribution. Drawing on an ecological study, the authors establish an association between the expansion of fast food restaurants and levels of obesity in their 26 country comparison. They therefore warn that the implication of trade liberalisation policies needs to be examined. The interaction between global, structural and personal factors is at the heart of food policy and its implications for public health. Chaufan, Fox and Hong's commentary provides a warning against policy which believes that simply labelling food outlet menus with calorie information will result in individual's making wiser choices. Moore et al.'s social-ecological approach suggests a way to combine macro- and micro-level factors and as such offers a route to examine the effectiveness at various points in the policy process. The evaluation offered by Law et al. of the livelihoods framework illustrates the need to focus upstream when considering policy. There are practical ways that, for example, supermarkets can act to enable its relatively poorer customers. De Vogli et al.'s findings also point to the need for an upstream focus. Although they are careful to stress the relationship between the availability of fast food restaurants and levels of obesity does not indicate causality, they reveal the association between global structural features and individual bodies. It is pertinent to be aware of the values underlying the conceptualisation of the problems being tackled as Pfeiffer et al. offer an insight into the construction of groups that may be the victims of 'collateral damage' (Bauman 2011) through the stigmatisation of obesity. Further, the increase in food prices had a predictably varied impact on different income groups in Dowler's study with 50% of households on below the relatively low income of £14,000 unable to afford the variety of food they were used to buying, compared with 20% of households on middle level incomes. Chaufan et al. call for public health stakeholders to more radically consider how to take poverty and other socio-economic determinants into account when developing food policy. The need to consider the dynamic interaction between the different levels in the policy process in order to ensure public health thus is apparent.

Article outlines

De Vogli et al. use the term 'globesization' to refer to the globalisation of the obesity epidemic. They locate this process in the inclusion of food markets in the promotion of worldwide free trade with the balance of power with transnational food companies. This is then a process that weakens public health interests. The evidence they use for illustration is the association between the density of the fast food company Subway in 26 high-income countries and levels of obesity. Although they caution against any suggestion of causality, they argue that more detailed investigation into this significant relationship is warranted. Trade policy cannot therefore be separated from public health and food policies.

Chaufan, Fox and Hong argue that interest in regulation to push food outlets to provide calorie information for consumers at the point of sale needs to consider the negative impact such a move could have. They say that whilst more individuals eat outside the home more often than in the past, there is little evidence that menu labelling will result in improved diets or a reduction in obesity rates or inequalities in health. Interest in menu labelling equates knowledge provision (calorie information) with an intended, positive outcome for whole populations (the consumption of fewer calories) without any consideration of the myriad of other factors which influence food and eating practices.

Dowler's contribution is located in concerns of volatility with a food system vulnerable to immediate as well as long-term, structural challenges. The study explores UK consumers' understanding of food security. This is a concept that has been developed in the context of low-income nations in order to assess access to appropriate food that is now being adopted more broadly. A proportion of UK consumers found increasing difficulty with such access due mainly to increases in food prices. The consequence of such a situation is the consumption of a greater proportion of low quality, less healthy food. While UK consumers equated the term food security with food safety, emphasising quality rather than access, they felt it was the government's responsibility to ensure both. Although they did not feel that the government was in a position to control food prices, it was nevertheless their role to ensure food was affordable. The findings emphasise the limited nature of consumer choice as a route to food and nutrition security.

Pfeiffer et al. argue in their study of German society that the focus on obesity is a way of hiding the real problem, which is hunger and nutritional poverty. Welfare policies contribute to nutritional poverty and social exclusion as the poor are unable to partake in taken for granted social activities such as eating out. Pfeiffer et al. demonstrate that in the context of neo-liberalism, the German state has delegated responsibility to protect people from hunger to the private and voluntary sector and thus reneged on its duty to safeguard the health of its population. In addition, obesity is stigmatised and assists with the marginalisation of the poor, serving as further evidence of their deficit in terms of lifestyle choice.

Chaufan et al. argue that the experience of 'being' poor impacts on food and other practices likely to influence the onset of diabetes among Latino communities in the USA. Their qualitative study of clients and service providers at a Non-Governmental Organisation clearly demonstrates that the barriers to eating healthily are related to the price of healthier foods; problems travelling to food outlets; the limitations of food assistance programmes; issues associated with immigration status; lack of employment /low pay and the need to juggle the requirement to eat with other aspects of daily living like needing to pay bills and maintain housing. The authors maintain that whatever participants' knowledge of or attitude towards eating healthily and avoiding diabetes, the experience of being poor makes it impossible to succeed at doing so. The authors argue for a radical rethink of public health policy to more fully acknowledge the lived reality of food insecurity.

Evans' study of how people manage food waste in England is located in the context of everyday practices and serves as a reminder that a focus at the consumer end has its limitations. There are many factors that contribute to food being wasted and as such emphasising the role of the individual over-estimates their ability to take action. Indeed, Evans argues that 'interventions might usefully be targeted at the social and material conditions in which food is provisioned'. The respondents in his study were conscious of reducing waste but many factors militated against success including the stress on healthy eating requiring fresh and therefore perishable food, food safety concerns, and work schedules as well as being sensitive to household preferences. Indeed, prioritising a reduction in waste demanded transgressing cultural boundaries of what constitutes a 'proper meal'.

Moore et al. make a case for the adoption of a social-ecological perspective in evaluating policy implementation and illustrates this with a case-study of primary school dining halls and their impact on children's healthy eating. This study, carried out in Wales, UK, is a good example of the complexity of implementing policy as this is never done in a vacuum. We see different issues emerging and Moore et al. identify ways of building an evidence base of effectiveness at every level. High-level policy, however well intentioned, is unlikely to be implemented in an effective manner unless the different steps taken in reaching the recipients are examined. Moore et al.'s case study illustrates the points where attention is required and evaluation may lead to improving the effectiveness of food policy for public health.

Law et al. examine the relevance of a livelihood framework, normally applied in developing countries, to data collected among single parent households in Australia. The framework is therefore 'imposed' on the interview data in order to assess its application in high-income countries. The framework includes the vulnerability context, individual livelihood capabilities and the transforming structures and processes. The findings indicate that the respondents possessed capabilities that could be better supported by structures and processes. The strength of the livelihood framework was the identification of potential policy interventions focused up-stream that would support individuals, such as regulation of food markets and supermarket pricing. However, the framework is less successful in acknowledging the sociocultural context; something that we have already noted is an important element to consider in public health nutrition yet remains a weakness in high-level policies.

Halkier and Jensen's study of the health interventions aimed at reducing type 2 diabetes and coronary heart disease among Pakistani Danes illustrates the problems of ignoring the socially and culturally embedded nature of eating. The respondents report on their interaction with diet advice to enhance health and avoid these common health problems. The advice offered became irrelevant as the food suggested as health inducing did not belong to the range of fare that the respondents would ordinarily eat. A focus on health was one of many considerations in the daily provision and consumption of food. Among the respondents' different social practices of 'doing food' were identified ranging from pro-active engagement with health as a priority to acknowledging that pleasure and care were primary aspects of food practices.

Milne also demonstrates the importance of being able to maintain daily food practices, here in order to limit risks to health from food poisoning. In his study of people over 60 years of age in England, there were clear points of vulnerability emerging as a result of changes to their everyday practices. Practical issues such as access to transport, shops and food storage were located in the cultural value system and experience of this generation. While food policy tends to separate food safety from nutrition, the changing food practices discussed among study participants point to their inter-relationship. The study further emphasised the need to create policies for rather than on the intended population.

Finally, Brembeck's study of the changing status of fish as a previously healthy, but now potentially dangerous, food in Sweden illustrates the tensions in protecting health and maintaining informed consumer choice. Located in theories of anxiety as social practice, this study identifies fears and anxiety as part of our collective experience. The role of the state as enabler of its citizens to manage the risks associated with fish consumption is clearly illustrated. The state has a supposedly unambiguous system for assessing and handling risks and then communicating this to consumers to enable them to make informed choices. Despite very clear messages, everyday life throws up considerable challenges for the young mothers in the study and a number of strategies for managing anxiety are required. Eating fish is not as simple as it may seem, especially if you are pregnant.

Conclusions

Food policy and its relationship to public health cover a multitude of intersecting issues. The papers in this collection highlight critiques relating to the lack of global regulation of the food supply chain and the predilection to leave this to markets and, in the end, to individual consumer decisions. Crucially, in these times of increased alarm with regard to sustainability, we also note the inadequate response to issues of waste, where solutions in high-income countries again are located to a large extent in lifestyle and consumer behaviour. The insight this collection of studies offers is the importance of considering everyday lived contexts in relation to policies on public health, food and sustainability. It is here that broader factors such as technological developments, ecological concerns and international trade are articulated and realised. The collection demonstrates the corrosive impact of social inequalities, and the futility of identifying poorer consumers as flawed, when aiming for food policies that seek to achieve positive public health.

References

Bauman, Z., 2011. Collateral damage: social inequalities in a global age. Cambridge, MA: Polity.

Caraher, M. and Coveney, J., 2003. Public health nutrition and food policy. Public Health Nutrition, 7 (5), 591–598.

Coveney, J., 2003. Why food policy is critical to public health. *Critical Public Health*, 13 (2), 99–105.

CSDH, 2008. Closing the gap in a generation: health equity through action on the social determinants of health. Final Report of the Commission on Social Determinants of Helat. Geneva: *World Health Organization.*

de Certeau, M., 1984. The practice of everyday life. S. Rendall, *trans.* Berkeley, CA: University of California Press.

Department of Health, 2010. Healthy lives, healthy people. Our strategy for public health in England. London: HMSO, CM7985.

Devisch, I. and Dierckz, K., 2009. On idiocy or the plea for an Aristotelian health policy. *Public Health*, 123, 514–516.

DFID, 2010. The neglected crisis of undernutrition: DFID's Strategy. London: Department for International Development.

Food Ethics Council, 2010. Food justice: the report of the food and fairness inquiry. London: The Food Ethics Council.

Foresight, 2011. The future of food and farming. Executive Summary. London: The Government Office for Science.

Green, J., 2010. The WHO Commission on Social Determinants of Health. *Critical Public Health*, 20 (1), 1–4.

Green, J. and Labonté, R., 2008. Critical perspectives in public health. London: Routledge.

Harris, J., et al., 2009. How food marketing contribute to childhood obesity and what can be done. *Annual Review of Public Health*, 30, 211–225.

Labonté, R., Frank, J., and Di Ruggiero, E., 2008. Introduction to unfair cases: social inequalities in health. In: J. Green and R. Labonté, eds. Critical perspectives in public health. London: Routledge, 13–78.

Lindsay, J., 2010. Health living guidelines and the disconnect with everyday life. *Critical Public Health*, 20 (4), 475–487.

Oxfam, 2011. Growing a better future. Food justice in a resource constrained world. Oxford: Oxfam GB.

Parfitt, J., Barthel, M., and Macnaughton, S., 2010. Food waste within food supply chains: quantification and potential for change to 2050. *The Royal Society*, 365, 3065–3081.

Poland, B. and Dooris, M., 2010. A green and healthy future: the settings approach to building health, equity and sustainability. *Critical Public Health*, 20 (3), 281–298.

Pottier, J., 1999. The anthropology of food. Cambridge, MA: Polity Press.

Tansey, G. and Rajotte, T., eds., 2008. The future control of food. London: Earthscan.

Thornley, L., Signal, L., and Thomson, G., 2010. Does industry regulation of food advertising protect child rights? *Critical Public Health*, 20 (1), 25–33.

van Rijnsoever, F., van Lente, H., and van Trijp, C., 2011. Systemic policies towards a healthier and more responsible food system. *Journal of Epidemiology and Community Health*, 65 (9), 737–739.

von Braun, J., 2011. Food price crises and health. Editorial. *British Medical Journal*, 342, 2474.

Wills, W., 2011. Introduction to food: representations and meanings, Special section on food. *Sociological Research* [online], 16 (2). Available from: http://www.socresonline.org.uk/16/2/16.html [Accessed 31 May 2011].

'Globesization': ecological evidence on the relationship between fast food outlets and obesity among 26 advanced economies

Roberto De Vogli[ab], Anne Kouvonen[c] and David Gimeno[d]

[a]Department of Health Behaviors and Health Education, School of Public Health, University of Michigan, Ann Arbor, MI 48109-2029, USA; [b]Department of Epidemiology and Public Health, International Institute for Society and Health, University College London, London, UK; [c]Warsaw School of Social Sciences and Humanities, Wroclaw Faculty, Wroclaw, Poland; [d]Division of Epidemiology, Human Genetics and Environmental Health Sciences, San Antonio Campus of the School of Public Health, The University of Texas Health Science Center at Houston, Houston, TX 77030, USA

The aim of this study was to investigate the relationship between the density of fast food restaurants and the prevalence of obesity by gender across affluent nations. Data on Subway's restaurants per 100,000 people and proportions of men and women aged 15 years or older with a body mass index higher or equal than $30 \, kg/m^2$ were obtained for 26 of 34 advanced economies. Countries with the highest density of Subway restaurants such as the USA (7.52 per 100,000) and Canada (7.43 per 100,000) also tend to have a higher prevalence of obesity in both men (31.3% and 23.2%, respectively) and women (33.2% and 22.9%, respectively). On the other hand, countries with a relatively low density of Subway restaurants such as Japan (0.13 per 100,000) and Norway (0.19 per 100,000) had a lower prevalence of obesity in both men (2.9% and 6.4%, respectively) and women (3.3% and 5.9%, respectively). Unadjusted linear regression models showed a significant correlation between the density of Subway's outlets and the prevalence of adult obesity ($\beta = 0.46$; $p = 0.02$ in men and $\beta = 0.48$; $p = 0.013$ in women). When the data were weighted by population size, the associations became substantially stronger in both men and women ($\beta = 0.85$; $p = 0.0001$ and $\beta = 0.84$; $p = 0.0001$, respectively). Covariate adjustment did not reduce the size of the associations. Our study raises serious concerns about the diffusion of fast food outlets worldwide and calls for coordinated political actions to address what we term 'globesization', the ongoing globalization of the obesity epidemic.

Introduction

Over the past 30 years, the prevalence of obesity has substantially increased in high-income countries (Yach *et al.* 2006). The diffusion of 'fast food restaurants' resulting from rapid global market integration (Hawkes 2009) and trade liberalization policies

(Thow and Hawkes 2009) seems to be one of the key contributing factors behind the sharp rise of obesity. Trade liberalization policies, in particular, have contributed to increase both exports of domestic goods and imports of foreign products and the opening of national markets to foreign investment. These reforms, strongly promoted by international financial institutions such as the World Trade Organization (WTO; Rayner *et al.* 2007) have been, and still are, particularly instrumental in promoting the growth and power of transnational food companies (TFCs; Hawkes 2009). The rising dominance and economic power of TFCs, the global spread of supermarkets and fast food companies such as McDonald's and Subway have produced dramatic changes in people's dietary patterns. A study by Bowman *et al.* (2004), for example, estimated that, in the USA, almost one-third of young people now eat at a fast food restaurant on any given day (Bowman *et al.* 2004). This can further increase the prevalence of obese and overweight adults in the future. A number of studies have, in fact, shown that consumption of items frequently sold in 'fast food' restaurants such as hamburgers and French fries is positively related with body weight (Jeffrey and French 1998, French *et al.* 2000, Prentice and Jebb 2003).

Although a growing number of studies have examined the association between the availability of fast food outlets and obesity (Fraser *et al.* 2010), only a few of them have analyzed the cross-national correlates of obesity (Rabin *et al.* 2007, Offer *et al.* 2010). In this article, we examined the association between the density of Subway's restaurants and the prevalence of obesity in men and women in 26 advanced economies. Subway is expected to overtake McDonald's as the world's largest fast-food chain in terms of outlets (Business-Week 2009).

Methods

Design and data sources

In order to study the relationship between the density of Subway's restaurants and the prevalence of obesity by gender in advanced economies, we conducted an ecological, cross-national study of countries with available data on both measures. Of the 34 advanced economies identified according to the International Monetary Fund (IMF 2009) criteria, data on obesity prevalence for men and women and on Subway restaurants were available for 26 countries. Data on the major dependent variable, obesity prevalence by gender (proportion of men and women aged ≥ 15 years with body mass index, BMI $\geq 30\,\mathrm{kg/m^2}$), were taken from the World Health Statistics (WHO 2009). The number of Subway's restaurants for each country was obtained from the Subway (Subway 2009) website as of December 2009. Population data for each advanced nation were used to calculate density measures of Subway's restaurants per 100,000 people. This measure was then transformed into a natural log indicator.

Covariates included a list of potential confounding factors that could explain the association between the density of fast food outlets and the prevalence of obesity. They included gross national income (GNI) per capita, proportion of people living in urban areas, the Gini coefficient, motor vehicles, and internet users. Data on GNI per capita (converted to international dollars using purchasing power parities), proportion of people living in urban areas, population size, motor vehicles per 1000 people, and internet users per 100 people were taken from the World Development

Indicators database published in 2009. Data on income inequality, measured by the Gini coefficient, were taken from the United Nations Development Program's Human Development Indicators published in 2009.

Statistical analyses

Unadjusted associations between the density of Subway restaurants and the prevalence of obesity separately for men and women were examined by simple linear regression models. Results of simple linear regression models are presented weighted and unweighted for population size. Multivariate linear regressions were used to calculate the standardized beta-coefficients (which equal the correlation coefficients, r) of the cross-national associations between Subway's restaurants per 100,000 people and the prevalence of obesity by gender controlling for covariates. A major concern for these multivariate analyses was the degree of multicollinearity between highly correlated predictors that could potentially result in unstable coefficients and standard errors. As an indicator of multicollinearity, we used variance inflation factor (VIF) values ≥ 10 (Belsley 1991). First, the associations of interest were adjusted for GNI per capita, urbanization and the Gini coefficient. A second model, where covariates also included motor vehicles per 1000 people and internet users per 100 people, presented problems of multicollinearity (VIF values for GNI per capita, the Gini coefficient and internet users were higher than 10). We therefore decided to drop the Gini coefficient from the model. Robust standard errors, the so-called 'sandwich estimators', were used to account for violations of the normality assumption in linear regressions (Baum 2006). Statistical analyses were conducted using Stata 11.0 software (StataCorp LP, College Station, TX).

Results

The results showed that there is a large variation in both the density of Subway's restaurants and the prevalence of obesity across the selected countries (Table 1). Countries with the highest density of Subway restaurants such as the USA (7.52 per 100,000) and Canada (7.43 per 100,000) also tend to have a higher prevalence of obesity in both men (31.3% and 23.2%, respectively) and women (33.2% and 22.9%, respectively). On the other hand, countries with a relatively low density of Subway restaurants such as Japan (0.13 per 100,000) and Norway (0.19 per 100,000) have a lower prevalence of obesity in both men (2.9% and 6.4%, respectively) and women (3.3% and 5.9%, respectively).

Scatterplots of data on the density of Subway's outlets and the prevalence of obesity in men and women across the 26 advanced economies are presented in Figure 1(a) and (b). Simple linear regression models showed that the density of Subway's outlets per 100,000 was significantly correlated with the prevalence of adult obesity in both genders ($\beta = 0.46$; $p = 0.02$ in men and $\beta = 0.48$; $p = 0.01$ in women). When the data were weighted by population size, the associations became substantially stronger in both men and women ($\beta = 0.85$; $p = 0.0001$ and $\beta = 0.84$; $p = 0.0001$, respectively). After adjustment for GNI per capita, urbanization and the Gini coefficient, the size of the associations remained strongly significant in both men ($\beta = 0.61$; $p = 0.001$) and women ($\beta = 0.57$; $p = 0.001$.). After additional adjustment for motor vehicles per 1000 people and internet users per 100 people

Table 1. The prevalence of obesity in men and women, the number of Subway restaurants per 100,000 and population size in 26 Advanced Economies, 2009.

Country	Percentage of people ≥15 years of age who are obese		Subway restaurants per 100,000	Population size (millions)
	Men	Women		
Australia	20.6	25.5	21.65	21.0
Austria	13.0	9.0	0.71	8.3
Belgium	11.9	13.4	0.15	10.4
Canada	23.2	22.9	7.43	33.2
Denmark	11.8	9.1	0.07	5.4
Finland	16.0	13.5	1.39	5.2
France	16.1	17.6	0.28	61.0
Germany	20.5	12.3	0.96	82.3
Greece	26.0	18.2	0.55	10.7
Iceland	12.4	12.3	5.91	0.3
Ireland	14.0	12.0	2.62	4.1
Israel	19.8	25.4	0.11	7.1
Italy	7.4	8.9	0.01	58.1
Japan	2.9	3.3	0.13	127.2
Netherlands	10.2	11.9	0.46	16.6
New Zealand	21.9	23.2	5.10	4.1
Norway	6.4	5.9	0.19	4.6
Portugal	15.0	13.4	0.01	10.6
Singapore	6.4	7.3	1.62	4.6
Slovakia	13.5	15.0	0.07	5.4
Spain	13.0	13.5	0.06	40.4
Sweden	11.0	9.5	0.69	9.0
Switzerland	7.9	7.5	0.05	7.5
UK	22.3	23.0	2.23	60.9
USA	31.3	33.2	7.52	303.8
Mean	14.8	14.6	1.59	33.9
SD	6.6	7.0	2.43	61.9

Notes: Hong Kong, Luxembourg, Malta, San Marino, Slovenia, South Korea and Taiwan were excluded because data on obesity prevalence were not available. Data for Austria came from WHO statistics (WHO 2009).

(excluding the Gini coefficient from the model to avoid problems of multi-collinearity), the associations still remained significant ($\beta = 0.72$; $p = 0.005$ and $\beta = 0.68$; $p = 0.002$).

Conclusions

The relationship between the density of fast food restaurants and the prevalence of obesity has received increasing attention in the literature. Several studies have shown that a higher density of fast food restaurants can be an environmental promoter of obesity (Jeffrey and French 1998, French et al. 2000, Prentice and Jebb 2003). Our findings indicate that the density of Subway's outlets is positively associated

(a)

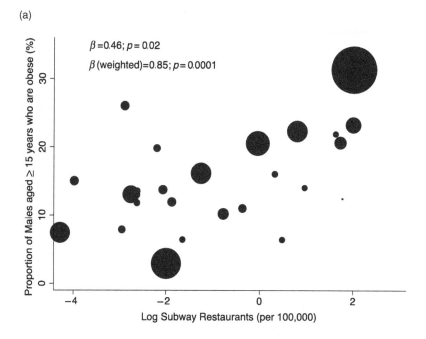

(b)

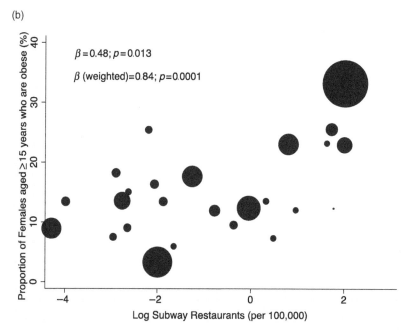

Figure 1. Subway restaurants per 100,000 people and prevalence of: (a) male obesity ($n = 26$) and (b) female obesity ($n = 26$) in advanced economies,[a] 2009.

Note: [a]List of countries includes Australia, Austria, Belgium, Canada, Czech Republic, Denmark, Finland, France, Germany, Greece, Iceland, Ireland, Israel, Italy, Japan, Netherlands, New Zealand, Norway, Portugal, Singapore, Slovakia, Spain, Sweden, Switzerland, United Kingdom and USA.

with the prevalence of obesity across 26 advanced economies in both men and women. These relationships remained significant after adjustment for GNI per capita, proportion of people living in urban areas and income inequality. They also remained significant in a model that included additional covariates such as motor vehicles per capita and internet users per capita.

Our results must be interpreted with caution. Given the cross-sectional study design, we cannot infer causality between the density of fast food restaurants and the prevalence of obesity. Also, the cross-sectional nature of our exploratory study does not take into account the potential time lag between exposure to fast food restaurants and the increase of obesity prevalence. Furthermore, our measure of the density of fast food outlets was restricted to only one fast food chain. Finally, although it is plausible to expect our findings to be relevant for middle- and low-income countries experiencing the 'nutrition transition' as well, our analysis were limited to adult populations of 26 advanced economies only. Data were not available for eight of the IMF advanced countries including large economies such as South Korea, Taiwan and Hong Kong: their exclusion may have influenced our results.

In spite of these shortcomings, our study provides novel findings of the ecological association between the availability of fast food and the prevalence of obesity in advanced economies. Our findings are consistent with aggregate level studies showing associations between fast food restaurants and obesity prevalence (Reidpath et al. 2002, Block et al. 2004, Maddock 2004, Cummins et al. 2005). An investigation of 50 US states showed that both the number of residents per fast food restaurant and the square miles per fast food restaurants were significantly associated with state-level obesity prevalence (Maddock 2004). In addition, a recent study showed that countries with market liberal welfare regimes (which are also English speaking) have a higher prevalence of obesity and easier access to fast food (e.g. a lower Big Mac relative price; Offer et al. 2010) than countries with different welfare regimes.

However, our results are inconsistent with findings at the individual level (Burdesse and Whitaker 2004, Jeffrey et al. 2006) showing no associations between proximity to fast food restaurants and obesity after adjustment for other factors. Some of these studies were affected by a number of shortcomings. One was restricted to low income children under the age of 5 years (Burdesse and Whitaker 2004). Another relied on self-reported measures of body height and weight and the frequency of eating at restaurants derived from a telephone survey (Jeffrey et al. 2006) that can be affected by self-report biases especially among low income groups. This is serious because evidence shows that people of low income are also more likely to be obese (Cummins et al. 2005). In a recent article, Fraser et al. argued that their review of studies investigating the relationship between availability to fast food outlets and overweight/obesity generated 'conflicting results'. The authors also specified that findings on the ecological associations between the density of fast food outlets and the prevalence of obesity 'have, largely, not been verified with the results from studies using individual level data' (Fraser et al. 2010). It is important to highlight, however, that the aim of ecological level analyses such as the one presented in this article is not to explain individual differences in obesity and increased access to fast food outlets, but societal level variations in environmental factors associated to obesity. The aim of aggregate level studies on the structural correlates of obesity is not to apply ecological level results to individuals and falling into the problem of 'ecological fallacy', (Pearce 2000) but to exclusively focus on policy-relevant, societal level determinants of health outcomes. Nevertheless, future policy-oriented research should investigate changes over time in obesity prevalence and the diffusion of fast food restaurants and trade liberalization policies across countries.

Finally, although our results are preliminary and exploratory, they suggest that the diffusion of fast food outlets, and trade liberalization policies promoting their growth and expansion worldwide, may contribute to the obesity epidemic. Our study also raises serious issues about the role of international financial institutions such as the WTO in promoting free trade and food market integration and calls for coordinated political actions to address what we term 'globesization', the ongoing globalization of the obesity epidemic.

Acknowledgments

RDV is supported by a grant from the Economic and Social Research Council (RES-070-27-0034), which is gratefully acknowledged.

References

Baum, C., 2006. *An introduction to modern econometrics using STATA*. College Station, TX: Stata Press.

Belsley, D., 1991. *Conditioning diagnostics: collinearity and weak data in regression*. New York, NY: Wiley.

Block, J., Scribner, R., and DeSalvo, K., 2004. Fast food, race/ethnicity and income: a geographical analysis. *American Journal of Preventive Medicine*, 27, 211–217.

Bowman, S., *et al.*, 2004. Effects of fast food consumption on energy intake and diet quality among children in a national household study. *Pediatrics*, 113, 112–118.

Burdesse, H. and Whitaker, R., 2004. Neighborhood playgrounds, fast food restaurants and crime: relationships to overweight in low-income preschool children. *Preventive Medicine*, 38, 57–63.

Business-Week, 2009. *Subway set to overtake McDonald's in store count*. Chicago, IL: Business Week.

Cummins, S., McKay, L., and McIntyre, S., 2005. McDonald's restaurants and neighborhood deprivation in Scotland and England. *American Journal of Preventive Medicine*, 29 (4), 308–310.

Fraser, L., *et al.*, 2010. The geography of fast food outlets: a review. *International Journal of Environmental Research and Public Health*, 7, 2290–2308.

French, S., Harnack, L., and Jeffrey, R., 2000. Fast food restaurant use among women in the Pound of prevention study: dietary, behavioural and demographic correlates. *International Journal of Obesity*, 24, 1353–1359.

Hawkes, C., 2009. Uneven dietary development: linking the policies and processes of globalization with the nutrition transition, obesity and diet-related chronic diseases. *Globalization and Health*, 2, 4.

IMF, 2009. *World economic outlook: crisis and recovery*. Washington, DC: International Monetary Fund.

Jeffrey, R. and French, S., 1998. Epidemic obesity in the United States: are fast foods and television viewing contributing? *American Journal of Public Health*, 88 (2), 277–280.

Jeffrey, R., *et al.*, 2006. Are fast food restaurants an environmental risk factor for obesity? *International Journal of Behavioural and Physical Activity*, 3, 2.

Maddock, J., 2004. The relationship between obesity and the prevalence of fast food restaurants: state-level analysis. *American Journal of Health Promotion*, 19 (2), 137–143.

Offer, A., Pechey, R., and Ulijaszek, S., 2010. Obesity under affluence varies by welfare regimes: the effect of fast food, insecurity, and inequality. *Economics and Human Biology*, 8 (3), 297–308.

Pearce, N., 2000. The ecological fallacy strikes back. *Journal of Epidemiology and Community Health*, 54, 326–327.

Prentice, A. and Jebb, S., 2003. Fast foods, energy density and obesity: a possible mechanistic link. *Obesity Reviews*, 4, 187–194.

Rabin, B., Boehmer, T., and Brownson, R., 2007. Cross-national comparison of environmental and policy correlates of obesity in Europe. *European Journal of Public Health*, 17 (1), 53–61.

Rayner, G., *et al.*, 2007. Trade liberalization and the diet transition: a public health response. *Health Promotion International*, 21 (S1), 67–73.

Reidpath, D., *et al.*, 2002. An ecological study of the relationship between social and environmental determinants of obesity. *Health and Place*, 8 (2), 141–145.

Subway, 2009. Official Subway Website. International Subway Locations. Available from: www.subway.com [Accessed 21 December 2009].

Thow, A. and Hawkes, C., 2009. The implications of trade liberalization for diet and health: a case study from Central America. *Globalization and Health*, 5, 5.

WHO, 2009. *World health statistics*. Geneva: World Health Organization.

Yach, D., Stuckler, D., and Brownell, K., 2006. Epidemiologic and economic consequences of the global epidemics of obesity and diabetes. *Nature Medicine*, 12 (1), 62–66.

Food for thought: menu labeling as obesity prevention public health policy

Claudia Chaufan, Patrick Fox and Gee Hee Hong

Department of Social & Behavioral Sciences, School of Nursing, Institute for Health & Aging, UC San Francisco, San Francisco, 94118 CA, USA

This article discusses the evidence for menu labeling as obesity prevention public health policy. While sympathetic to providing nutritional information, whether food is consumed at restaurants or purchased for home consumption, the authors raise a word of caution against the assumption that menu labeling will significantly lead to healthier food choices, lower obesity rates, and decreased obesity disparities. The authors find little empirical evidence that this will be the case, critique the theoretical model that informs menu labeling as obesity prevention public health policy, and instead encourage policies that draw on a fundamental social causes approach to obesity prevention and health promotion generally.

Introduction

Over the past decade, the public perception of obesity has shifted from considering it a character flaw to recognizing it as a problem with complex societal roots and embedded in toxic environments. An intervention alleged to improve such environments that has received broad support is mandating that restaurants provide information about the nutritional content of their menus (hereafter, menu labeling).

In this commentary, we raise a word of caution against the current enthusiasm for menu labeling as obesity prevention policy. We do not deny that relative excess calories cause obesity, nor are we unsympathetic in informing consumers about the nutritional, especially caloric, content of food items, and we grant that individuals may want, or have a right to know this information. Yet faced with rising obesity rates and with the fact that obesity stubbornly remains an unequal opportunity disease, even as the nutritional information available to consumers has increased dramatically since the Nutrition Labeling and Education Act of 1990 (NLEA), we conclude that menu labeling will do little to reduce the obesity rates, much less inequalities in their distribution, and may ultimately hinder the public understanding of the epidemic.

Adequate responses to obesity and related conditions require sociologically grounded models of health and disease, and we encourage one such model, if the goal is to develop successful obesity prevention and health promotion generally.

The rationale for menu labeling

Support for menu labeling builds on the observation that over the few decades, residents in industrialized economies increasingly rely on eating out (Berman and Lavizzo-Mourey 2008) and that food prepared away from home, especially from fast-food restaurants, is greater in calories than home-made food (Jeffery and French 1998). Surveys conducted by the US Department of Agriculture reveal that between 1977–1978 and 1994–1996, the daily calorie intake from food away from home increased from 18% to 32% (Variyam 2006). Similarly, in 2004, the Office for National Statistics in the UK estimated that spending on eating out had doubled since 1992 (Mesure 2006).

Vis-à-vis this state of affairs, the American Public Health Association (APHA) has enthusiastically endorsed menu labeling as 'a critical step in combating the growing obesity epidemic and encouraging healthier habits' (American Public Health Association 2009, p. 2), US legislators working feverishly to pass health care reform have included a menu labeling provision that would mandate chain restaurants to display the calorie content of each standard menu item publicly (Senate Committe on Health, Labor and Pensions 2009), and since July 2008, over 15 food outlets in New York City have been required to post the caloric content of their dishes (Barron 2008). The enthusiasm for menu labeling as obesity prevention policy is not limited to the United States alone. Already in January of 2008, the European Commission was considering enacting menu labeling legislation for the 27-country bloc to fight the rising obesity rates (Bounds et al. 2008).

This enthusiasm for informing the public about the nutritional content of food items in order to encourage healthier eating habits is not new: the NLEA was hailed by the then US Secretary of Health and Human Services, Dr. Louis Sullivan, as legislation that would allow consumers to 'use a single format for virtually all processed foods to compare nutrition values and make healthy choices' (U.S. Department of Health and Human Services 1992). In this spirit, obesity experts Ludwig and Brownell recently underscored the strengths of menu labeling, arguing that it can abate what economists call 'asymmetric information' between consumers and marketers of food so a better informed public would make healthier food choices that would in turn lead to lower obesity rates, that it has the capacity to enhance the effect of public health campaigns encouraging individuals to make healthier food choices, and that changes in consumption patterns could in turn provide incentives for restaurants to increase the supply of healthier options, in response to their increased demand (Ludwig and Brownell 2009).

Problematic premises

Notwithstanding the excitement for menu labeling among experts and policy makers, the trouble is that there is little evidence for its *actual* effectiveness, and good reasons to believe that it reflects an overly simplistic view of obesity, of human health, and of health inequalities more generally. To begin with, body weight is not only the product of calories intake relative to expenditure, but also of a life-long developmental process, beginning as early as the fetal stage where behaviors play little, if any, role (Benyshek 2007), and sensitive to multiple social determinants that severely limit access to resources necessary for health among socially excluded groups (Benyshek 2007, Chaufan and Weitz 2009).

Menu labeling addresses one aspect of the problem, calorie intake when eating out, and assumes that disclosing nutritional information at restaurants offering foods of generally high fat and calorie content will lead consumers to healthier choices in those occasions, thus to lower weights. Nonetheless, the question remains: 'would consumers with perfect, or improved nutritional information make healthier food choices?' The answer depends on many variables. For instance, some individuals prioritize taste above other factors and avoid foods dubbed as 'healthy' assuming they are less palatable (O'Dougherty *et al.* 2006). In addition, even when nutritional information and the convenience of healthier choices are understood, these may be unaffordable. Such was the case of a recent study in low-income neighborhoods, where menu labeling made no difference to *actual* calorie intake, even if individuals *claimed* that the intervention influenced their choices (Elbel *et al.* 2009).

Additionally, menu labeling may have unintended and undesirable effects, as illustrated by a recent food-labeling campaign in the United States, *Smart Choices*, designed as a 'nutrition labeling program [that] helps shoppers make smarter food and beverage choices within product categories in every supermarket aisle' (Neuman 2009). As the campaign was launched, it gave its sign of approval, a green check mark of a 'smart choice', to *Froot Loops*, a sugar-laden cereal marketed to children, that the chairman of the nutrition department of the Harvard School of Public Health referred to as a 'horrible' choice (Neuman 2009).

While the campaign could have been dismissed as a purely commercial initiative, promoting corporate rather than public interests, it was not. Rather, it was enthusiastically endorsed by the doctors affiliated with prestigious academic and professional institutions, such as Tufts University, Baylor College of Medicine, the American Diabetes Association, and the American Dietetic Association (Beck 2009), who argued that breakfast cereals such as Froot Loops were after all a 'better choice' than a doughnut (Neuman 2009). Some of these doctors, but not all, recanted after Change.org, a grassroots organization, denounced 'the Smart Choices Ploy', which was finally called off after a petition drew thousands of signatures from angry citizens, and a member of the US House of Representatives urged the Food and Drug Administration to launch an investigation on the program (Beck 2009, DeLauro calls investigation, 2009).

Yet another problematic dimension of nutrition labels is their intelligibility. For instance, packaged food producers are required to display information 'per serving', and information about total calories-per-serving is clearly critical to the success of menu labeling as obesity prevention policy. Yet what counts as 'one serving' in a label does not necessarily coincide with the common understanding of a serving. For instance, one Reese's Brownie contains 380 calories. Yet the package label displays the calorie information of one *half* brownie, considered 'one serving.' While most people can figure out that, if they eat one brownie, they should multiply 190 by 2 to estimate the total calorie content, unless they are already *alert* that a serving in the label is not necessarily a serving as they usually think of; they will end up consuming more calories than what they anticipate.

Finally, and most critically, menu labeling fails to address the skewed distribution of obesity, vastly more prevalent among the poor, for well-studied reasons that increase individuals' exposure to unhealthier environments and lifestyles (Gordon-Larsen *et al.* 2006, Simon *et al.* 2008). Granted that factors *other* than nutritional information influence food choices does not *in itself* speak *against* menu labeling, yet lack of evidence for its effectiveness warns against the current enthusiasm and suggests that answers to the epidemic may lie elsewhere.

What to do

Over 200 years of anecdotal, epidemiological, and experimental evidence indicate that living conditions are causally related to the distribution of disease, even as the major types of diseases and the particular mechanisms linking those conditions with disease have changed over time (Link and Phelan 1995, Raphael 2007). Early study in the traditions of public health and social epidemiology led medical researchers and practitioners such as Rudolf Virchow to suggest that the best way to reduce disease was to improve the living conditions and increase the political power of the poor (Waitzkin 1981). A modern incarnation of this tradition is Link and Phelan's theory of 'fundamental social causes' of health and disease (Link and Phelan 1995). This approach to understand the determinants of health and, importantly, of health inequalities, proposes that across time and diseases, social power – in the form of money, knowledge, prestige, and beneficial social connections – allows better-off individuals to protect or restore their health by utilizing whatever resources are available in that time and place (Link and Phelan 1995).

So in the spirit of the forefathers of public health, the theory predicts that health inequalities will be greater for curable or highly preventable diseases, such as pneumonia, lower for non-curable diseases, such as pancreatic cancer, and minimal to non-existent for conditions that are inevitable, such as death after a person reaches a very late age, which is precisely the case (Phelan and Link 2005). Likewise with obesity, a highly preventable condition (Benyshek 2007), for which the theory predicts that the greater the inequalities in social power, the greater the social inequalities in its distribution will be. And this is also the case, both in developed and developing countries, where obesity disproportionately affects minorities and the poor (Sobal and Stunkard 1989, Monteiro *et al.* 2004).

It follows that if menu labeling effectively reduced information asymmetry between the 'average consumer' and an increasingly powerful food industry, which we doubt for the reasons offered so far, it would also have the unintended effect of increasing, rather than decreasing, inequalities in the distribution of obesity, by increasing the power gap (to take care of one's health in the multiple known ways) between the haves and the have-nots.

Fortunately for prevention, it also follows that policies that reduce socioeconomic inequalities (such as mandating living wages), or that at least improve access to healthier food and exercise environments for socially excluded groups, should lead to more sustainable changes in obesity rates and reduction of inequalities in obesity (and in health, more generally) than those premised on a purely 'informational' view of human behavior and human health (Navarro and Shi 2001). Such interventions include subsidizing healthier food options through farmers' markets, school lunch programs, or worksite cafeterias, providing economic incentives to businesses offering these options in low-income neighborhoods, and investing on healthier built environments (Chaufan *et al.* 2009). Measures could be partly financed through taxes on consumer goods known to have an unfavorable impact on health, such as sodas (Brownell and Frieden 2009).

Over the last decades, American society has become increasingly unequal, with stagnating wages even as workers' productivity and corporate profits have grown (Baker 2007). This has also been the case in other wealthy societies, such as the United Kingdom (Office for National Statistics 2009) and Canada (Raphael 2007). The critical question is how much poverty and social inequality societies are willing to tolerate, which will translate into the amount of obesity and obesity inequalities, among other deteriorating health indices, they will have to tolerate as well. We contend that any evidence-based obesity prevention public health policy should take the relationship between obesity and socioeconomic inequality seriously, and that policies tending to minimize these inequalities, or short of this, their impact, offer the greatest potential to improve food choices, reduce obesity and obesity inequalities, and promote better health.

References

American Public Health Association, 2009. *APHA supports menu labeling proposal*, in *The Nation's Health*. Washington, DC: APHA, 2.

Baker, D., 2007. *Behind the gap between productivity and wage growth*. Washington, DC: Center for Economic and Policy Research. Available from: http://www.cepr.net/documents/publications/0702_productivity.pdf [Accessed 15 September 2009].

Barron, J., 2008. *Restaurants must post calories, judge affirms*, in *The New York Times*. New York. Available from: http://www.nytimes.com/2008/04/17/nyregion/17calorie.html [Accessed 17 April 2008].

Beck, R., 2009. *Change.org activists get health organizations to back away from 'Smart Choices' food labeling ploy*. Change.org. Available from: http://food.change.org/blog/view/changeorg_activists_get_health_organizations_to_back_away_from_smart_choices_food_labeling_ploy [Accessed 15 September 2009].

Benyshek, D.C., 2007. The developmental origins of obesity and related health care disorders: prenatal and perinatal factors. *Collegium Antropologicum*, 31 (1), 315–319.

Berman, M. and Lavizzo-Mourey, R., 2008. Obesity prevention in the information age: caloric information at the point of purchase. *The Journal of the American Medical Association*, 300 (4), 433–435.

Bounds, A., Tait, N., and Wiggins, J., EU proposes food label rules. *Financial Times*, 31 January 2008, London, World News, p. 4.

Brownell, K.D. and Frieden, T.R., 2009. Ounces of prevention – the public policy case for taxes on sugared beverages. *The New England Journal of Medicine*, 360 (18), 1805–1808.

Chaufan, C., Hong, G.H., and Fox, P., 2009. Economic perspectives on public health policies to reduce obesity in california, commissioned by the California Department of Public Health. Unpublished, 1–90.

Chaufan, C. and Weitz, R., 2009. The elephant in the room: the invisibility of poverty in research on type 2 diabetes. *Humanity and Society*, 33, 74–98.

DeLauro calls investigation, 2009. *DeLauro calls for fda investigation into 'Smart Choice' labeling urges reclassification of froot loops, other sugary cereals*, 21 September 2009. Available from: http://delauro.house.gov/release.cfm?id = 2653 [Accessed 22 September 2009].

Elbel, B., *et al.*, 2009. Calorie labeling and food choices: a first look at the effects on low-income people in New York city. *Health Affairs*, 28 (6), 1110–1121.

Gordon-Larsen, P., *et al.*, 2006. Inequality in the built environment underlies key health disparities in physical activity and obesity. *Pediatrics*, 117 (2), 417–424.

Jeffery, R.W. and French, S.A., 1998. Epidemic obesity in the United States: are fast foods and television viewing contributing? *American Journal of Public Health*, 88 (2), 277–280.

Link, B. and Phelan, J., 1995. Social conditions as fundamental causes of disease. *Journal of Health and Social Behavior*, 35, 80–94.

Ludwig, D.S. and Brownell, K.D., 2009. Public health action amid scientific uncertainty: the case of restaurant calorie labeling regulations. *The Journal of the American Medical Association*, 302 (4), 434–435.

Mesure, S., 2006. *Britain spending more on eating out than dining at home, in The Independent.* 19 August 2006. Available from: http://license.icopyright.net/user/viewFree Use.act?fuid = NzMxOTYyNw%3D%3D [Accessed 19 February 2010].

Monteiro, C.A., *et al.*, 2004. Socioeconomic status and obesity in adult populations of developing countries: a review. *Bulletin of the World Health Organization*, 82 (12), 940–946.

Navarro, V. and Shi, L., 2001. The political context of social inequalities in health. *Social Science and Medicine*, 52, 481–491.

Neuman, W., 2009. For your health, froot loops. *The New York Times*, Saturday, 5 September, New York, B1–B5.

O'Dougherty, M., *et al.*, 2006. Nutrition labeling and value size pricing at fast-food restaurants: a consumer perspective. *American Journal of Health Promotion*, 20 (4), 247–250.

Office for National Statistics, 2009, *Income: gaps in income and wealth remain large.* Available from: http://www.statistics.gov.uk/cci/nugget.asp?id = 1005 [Accessed 9 November].

Phelan, J. and Link, B., 2005. Controlling disease and creating disparities: a fundamental cause perspective. *The Journal of Gerontology*, 60B (Special Issue II), 27–33.

Raphael, D., 2007. *Poverty and policy in Canada.* Toronto: Canadian Scholars' Press.

Senate Committe on Health, Labor and Pensions, 2009. *America's Affordable Health Choices Act.* July 15 2009. Available from: http://mikulski.senate.gov/NewsLinks/HealthReform/ AffordableHealthChoicesActSummary.pdf [Accessed 15 August 2009].

Simon, P.A., *et al.*, 2008. Proximity of fast food restaurants to schools: do neighborhood income and type of school matter? *Preventive Medicine*, 47 (3), 284–288.

Sobal, J. and Stunkard, A., 1989. Socioeconomic status and obesity: a review of the literature. *Psychological Bulletin*, 105 (2), 260–276.

U.S. Department of Health and Human Services, 1992. *Regulation – labeling for processed foods – press release.* Available from: http://www.hhs.gov/news/press/pre1995pres/ 921202.txt [Accessed 20 April 2009].

Variyam, J.N., 2006. *Nutrition labeling in the food-away-from-home sector: an economic assessment (a report from the economic research service).* Washington, DC: United States Department of Agriculture – USDA. Available from: http://www.ers.usda.gov/publications/ err4/err4.pdf [Accessed 6 April 2009].

Waitzkin, H., 1981. The social origins of illness: a neglected history. *International Journal of Health Services*, 11, 77–103.

Thinking about 'food security': engaging with UK consumers

Elizabeth A. Dowler[a], Moya Kneafsey[b], Hannah Lambie[c], Alex Inman[d] and Rosemary Collier[e]

[a]Department of Sociology, University of Warwick, Coventry CV4 7AL, UK; [b]Department of Geography, Environment and Disaster Management, Coventry University, Coventry CV1 5FB, UK; [c]Applied Research Centre in Sustainable Regeneration, Futures Institute, Coventry University Technology Park, Coventry CV1 2TL, UK; [d]Alex Inman Consulting, Launceston, Cornwall PL15 9SL, UK; [e]Crop Research Centre, School of Life Sciences, University of Warwick, Coventry CV4 7AL, UK

'Food security' has recently gained policy salience in the UK and internationally. Definitions vary, but the term is generally used by policy makers to imply sustained access by all consumers to sufficient food that is affordable, safe, nutritious and appropriate for an active and healthy life. Recent attention partly reflects anxiety over possible resource and environmental instabilities within the food system and the effects of economic recession. Food prices are often used to signal potential food insecurity; prices have risen recently in Britain as elsewhere, along with increased fuel costs and significant financial and job insecurities. All these factors are likely to have differential effects on food management in households living in different social and economic circumstances. Recent research using a mixed methods approach explored some of these complexities by engaging with UK consumers to examine people's reactions to increasing food prices and their views on responsibility for 'food security'. Well aware of increased food costs, most could identify key commodities and many cited increased oil and input prices as causes; some made links to the larger financial crisis. Few knew the term 'food security'; though most initially interpreted it as food safety and quality, the idea that affordable, healthy food should be available and accessible for all was widely recognised. Many saw this as increasingly difficult for themselves and others in current circumstances and, while acknowledging commercial realities, look to government primarily to secure nutrition and food security for all.

Introduction

Reliable access to and regular consumption of healthy food is recognised as an essential social determinant of health and public health policy has a long history of involvement in assuring its continuity for the general population. The contemporary food system broadly ensures provision of food of consistent quality and relative cheapness for ever increasing populations through technological, scientific and management advances, although substantial numbers are still too poor to obtain, grow or rear enough food to avoid hunger and malnutrition (FAO 2009). Nevertheless, growing challenges to the environmental and social sustainability and concentration of power are emerging (Roberts 2008, Godfray et al. 2010), and, in its quest for driving down costs to consumers, the food system is accused of failing to support nutritional health and well-being (Patel 2007, Lang et al. 2009). Despite movements towards new ways of engaging with the food system, partly out of reaction to these problems (Maye et al. 2007, Kneafsey et al. 2008), few among the general public in Europe are fully aware of expert anxieties or the concomitant re-emergence of ideas about 'food security' at international, national and household levels. This article draws on recent mixed method research in the UK, employing a 1000 sample online quantitative questionnaire and 15 deliberative qualitative workshops in urban and rural areas of the West and East Midlands and South West. We first briefly outline the context of rising food prices and emerging discourses on 'food security', before exploring the general public's reactions to the former, and understanding of the latter, and responsibility for its maintenance.

The background to the research was the recent vulnerabilities of the international food system to short-term shocks as well as to longer term challenges. For the former, the global food price spike of 2007–2008 triggered considerable anxiety internationally about civil unrest and provoked re-emergence of concern over the security of food supply and access, at global and national levels. The reasons why prices rose as fast and as suddenly as they did and remained volatile since have been much debated (Evans 2008, von Braun 2008, Global Foods Market Group undated) and probably include systemic factors such as rising oil costs (with significant impact on industrialised farming); droughts in grain-producing nations reducing world stockpiles; possibly increased use of crops for biofuel; possibly growing international demand for meat; and almost certainly the collapse of the sub-prime market and thus increased commodity speculation in financial markets (de Schutter 2010). As a result, the United Nations convened a High-Level Task Force (HLTF) in 2008 to coordinate analysis and response (HLTF 2008) and international meetings and reports (FAO 2009) have been echoed at national levels (for instance, in the UK, The Strategy Unit (2008) and Ambler-Edwards et al. (2009)). Longer term concerns about food system sustainability have focused on the current and future impacts of climate change, the end of affordable fossil fuel based energy and global population growth. A major collaborative international report presenting radical, agro-ecological approaches (IAASTD 2008), has been followed in the UK by the recent Foresight Report, also international in scope, which is rather more focused on technological solutions (Foresight 2011). In all these, the seeming intractability of continuing food inequality and malnutrition are also discussed.

Since the UK food system is based primarily on industrialised agriculture and internationally traded foodstuffs, it is vulnerable to the same forces producing shocks as elsewhere, with similar results. In particular, the price of basic UK food commodities and products rose sharply in 2007, and, although the supermarkets kept prices as low as they could – indeed, several compete on low price – the year-on-year decline in relative food price seen since the late 1990s has not returned. Despite some fluctuations and periods of stability, broadly speaking, the price of many foods remained higher in mid-2010 than pre-2007. (For instance, eggs were 46% higher, butter 43%, cheese 27%, milk 26%, beef 23%, bread 22% and poultry 17%, although the relative prices of fruit and vegetables declined slightly [Defra 2010; Department for Environment, Food and Rural Affairs, Defra]). Considerable concern has been expressed in the media and by the voluntary sector over the consequences for people, in general, and lower income households, in particular, since energy costs were also rising and wages and state benefits were not increasing commensurately. Charitable foodbanks report rising usage (Trussell Trust website http://www.trusselltrust.org/foodbank-projects) by those needing emergency food help.

Food security

A renewed discourse of 'food security' has emerged, internationally and in the UK, though not without contestation (Patel 2009, MacMillan and Dowler 2011); such a notion has a long history and reach (Maxwell 1996). Space precludes elaborate account here (see Maxwell (2001) and Shaw (2007) among many) but note that early formulation during the 1974 World Food Council in response to production crises and price spikes was rapidly construed as also critical in reducing international hunger and malnutrition. Subsequently, ideas about access (economic and spatial) as well as appropriateness of food were introduced, with an emphasis on accessing enough food to live an active, healthy life (FAO 1996). Critical paradigm shifts in approach have been from global to national, household and individual focus; from a perspective on food as primary need to one where livelihood security is seen as key; and from objective to subjective indicators as legitimate sources of causal analysis and policy response (Maxwell 1996, 2001). Until recently, however, with the exception of the US which has long used household food security indicators to identify households in need of food welfare intervention (Nord *et al.* 2010), most rich countries' governments regarded 'food security' as a concern confined to the global south. Certainly, within the UK, household food security played no part in policy formulation until the last few years, although the concept was used, for instance, by a poverty NGO in Scotland to engage local-level practitioners and household members in discussions over problematics of the food system (Killeen 2000). However, food price instabilities and concern over food system social and environmental sustainability have meant 'food security' has become legitimate policy focus in the UK (MacMillan and Dowler 2011), and the definition adopted by Defra in 2006 drew on FAO (1996) as: 'Food security exists when all people, at all times, have physical and economic access to sufficient, safe and nutritious food to meet their dietary needs and food preferences for an active and healthy life' (Defra 2006, p. 81). The essential mechanisms for ensuring all have access to food in the UK remain: operation of efficient markets in retail and employment, appropriate consumer choice and a social welfare system which is meant to enable those lacking employment to be able to purchase food. There are echoes in contemporary public health policy in England, which under 'Change4life' (Department of Health 2010) employs a social marketing approach to changing food behaviour, in partnership with the private sector. In practice, neither Defra nor the Department of Health has, nor ever has had, the responsibility for ensuring that household have sufficient income available for food purchase to fulfil their food and nutrition security needs (although the latter housed the Welfare Food Scheme and now manages 'Healthy Start', a food benefit targeted at low-income mothers of young children) (Dowler 2002). In fact, during 2010, there was growing evidence that increasing numbers of households in the UK were unlikely to be able to afford enough safe, nutritious food to meet current guidelines for healthy living (Dowler 2010) because they had insufficient 'economic access' to be food secure. 'Consumer choice' has long been criticised as an effective mechanism for ensuring appropriate food purchase and intake, particularly for those on lower incomes and/or living in areas of multiple deprivation where spatial and economic access to sufficient affordable food for a healthy life can be very difficult (Dowler *et al.* 2007, Lang *et al.* 2009, among many).

While 'food security' has gained an increasingly significant profile in both academic and policy circles, its connection to public health and what has come to be termed 'nutrition security' has been less evident. WHO argues, in its 2000 Plan for Action over food and diet for Europe, that nutrition security in the twenty-first century depends on production which meets dietary needs, more equal access to appropriate food and control of misleading promotional messages (Robertson *et al.* 2004), yet few of these elements is evident in agriculture, food or health policies in the UK or in many other European countries. Furthermore, little research has been done into what the general public, whether constructed as economic agents (consumers or shoppers), or as recipients of health promotional activities to encourage or enable eating behaviours closer to recommended practice, think about 'food security'. This then was the purpose of this research, undertaken during 2009–2010, against the background of rising food prices and general concerns over food system sustainability, as well as rising levels of obesity.

Investigating consumers' views: aims and methods

The overall aim was to assess UK consumers' understanding of, and reactions to, changing food prices and food security and their expectations of government and other actors in the food system. The empirical research, commissioned by Defra, was carried out between July 2009 and July 2010 and used a sequential mixed methodological approach, involving an online quantitative survey and a series of qualitative, deliberative workshops, with consumers who self-identified as 'primary shoppers'. The aim of the quantitative phase was to identify trends in consumer behaviour in relation to food price increases and preliminary views of food security in relation to broad socio-economic and demographic differentials. The qualitative phase built on the understanding gained to explore in-depth thinking about, and responses to, rising food prices and to engage with people's understanding of and reactions to notions of 'food security'.

An online survey method was used in order to obtain reasonable response rates; face-to-face interviewing was ruled out because of time and costs (Braunsberger *et al.* 2007). A stratified, random sample of the NOP-GfK (http://www.gfknop.com/) Consumer Panel was recruited; this panel is itself randomly recruited on an ongoing basis, to take part in consumer research. The panel includes adults aged 18 and over from all key socio-economic cohorts, including low-income groups; people are asked to identify which of the 10 income bands their household occupied; 8% of the total panel population households earn below £7000 p.a. and 13% between £7000 and £14,000 p.a. The sample for the study was proportionally stratified (using quotas) to be representative of the 18+ primary food purchaser population across several socio-demographic variables, specifically, gender, age, household income, car ownership, household size and geographical location. The unit of analysis was the individual respondent, but the questionnaire, designed by the authors and administered via GfK NOP, obtained data on household purchasing and decision making. It was administered through a secure website, contained 41 questions (including some open-ended answers) and took around 25 min to complete. Data collection and analysis were carried out in full accordance with the Data Protection Act and the Market Research Society's Code of Conduct to guarantee respondent confidentiality; the questionnaire received approval both from Defra Survey Control Unit and the relevant University ethical committee.

Just over 1000 questionnaires were completed (no refusals); there were slightly more in the lower income groups than in the total panel (23% between £7000 and £14,000 p.a.). Rapid cross-tabulation analysis of the questionnaire results informed the design of the qualitative research phase, which was a series of deliberative workshops with participants recruited in terms of key demographic, life stage and household criteria thought likely to influence attitudes and behaviours towards components of 'food security' (access, affordability and availability). The sampling strategy was therefore organised first around household income, having dependent children, single households or by location, all factors which the survey had confirmed as relevant to experiencing food insecurity, including those who had recently experienced income change through job loss. Second, to satisfy Defra's needs, some workshops were recruited around characteristics Defra had identified in an earlier work which segmented populations in terms of views, values and intentions towards environmental problems (Defra 2008). Where possible, women only and 'all-white' groups, were avoided.

In total, 15 workshops were run by the authors with main food shoppers, in urban and rural locations in the West and East Midlands and the South West; they involved simple group activities and facilitated discussions. All discussions were taped and videoed (for checking purposes only); tapes were transcribed and explored using thematic analysis.

Survey and workshop results

Table 1 gives the breakdown of the online survey sample in terms of socio-demographic characteristics in relation to the panel sample; these are broadly characteristic of the UK population, although the sample has more low-income consumers, with about a fifth having no car access. For about a quarter, household income had decreased in the previous 2 years, and around a half said their income had remained about the same. When asked about food expenditure, 12% said they spent under £100/month, 31% £100–£200; 38% £201–£400; and 13% over £400. Although these data represent quick expenditure estimates, the results are reasonably typical of UK spending patterns (in 2009, the lowest decile spent just over £100/month, and the top decile about £340 a month, on food [ONS 2010]); spending on food may have, of necessity, fallen since 2009, as the cost of other household essentials rose.

Table 1. Online survey respondents: socio-demographic characteristics of achieved sample in relation to panel population.

	18 + Primary purchaser population (%)	Achieved sample profile (%)		18 + Primary purchaser population (%)	Achieved sample profile (%)
Gender			*Car ownership*		
Female	66	64	Yes	72	80
Male	34	36	No	28	20
Age			*Number of people in household*		
18–24	9	9	1	26	27
25–34	16	16	2	33	34
35–44	20	21	3	18	18
45–54	17	18	4	15	15
55–64	16	16	5+	8	6
65+	22	20			
Household income			*Country*		
Up to £14,000	33	30	England	83	83
£14,001 to £28,000	23	25	Scotland	9	9
£28,001 to £48,000	29	30	Wales	5	5
£48,001+	15	15	North Ireland	3	3

Food prices: access and affordability

Perhaps unsurprisingly, 90% of consumers in the online survey had noticed food prices rising over the previous 2 years, 50% saying they had 'increased a lot', and, in common with all workshop participants, most noticeable price increases were for bread, dairy and meat, whichever income bracket or social group they came from. In the online survey, 37% said they were finding it more difficult to afford the variety of food they wanted to buy, a proportion which varied by income group: it was 50% for households with income below £14,000 and only 20% for those with income > £41,000.[1] Indeed, about a fifth of online respondents considered the cost of food to be a serious source of stress for themselves and their families; this proportion doubled if respondents were from the lowest income group and/or households with children. Of those noting increasing food prices, 57% had had to make savings on other household items or activities to manage their expenditures; this proportion again varied by income group and presence of children (for instance, only 36% had cut other expenditure to buy food if their income exceeded £41,000). People had cut back in buying clothes and holidays, and nearly three quarters of those making savings were less frequently eating out of the home (Figure 1). Almost a third said they had reduced heating or electricity consumption to meet food bills, a proportion which rose to 40% in lower income groups ($p = 0.016$). People had adjusted buying habits in various ways: they tried to bulk buy, hunted for bargains or supermarket 'own brands' and nearly two-thirds mentioned throwing less food away; all such strategies were more likely to be mentioned by lower income households. Nearly a fifth of respondents with children said they (adults) regularly went without food to ensure their children received enough to eat.

29

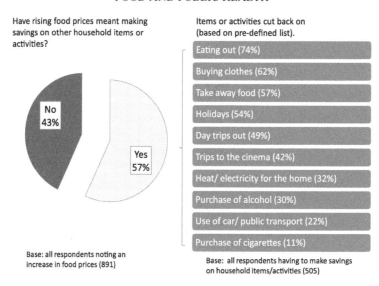

Have rising food prices meant making savings on other household items or activities?

No 43%

Yes 57%

Base: all respondents noting an increase in food prices (891)

Items or activities cut back on (based on pre-defined list).

Eating out (74%)

Buying clothes (62%)

Take away food (57%)

Holidays (54%)

Day trips out (49%)

Trips to the cinema (42%)

Heat/ electricity for the home (32%)

Purchase of alcohol (30%)

Use of car/ public transport (22%)

Purchase of cigarettes (11%)

Base: all respondents having to make savings on household items/activities (505)

Figure 1. Survey responses: reactions to rising food prices.

Similar comments were made by workshop participants. Several people drew on personal stories of living on restricted incomes, either long term or because of loss of a job, giving detailed accounts of the range of strategies. All spent time looking for bargains, supermarket 'own brands' and special offers; some had switched to using discount chains or local markets. People explained strategies for throwing less away (freezing leftovers and portions from bulk cooking) and reducing meat consumption; many emphasised cooking from ingredients rather than buying ready-made, more expensive, products. For some, feeding themselves and their family was a continual struggle, which they found difficult to articulate even if they were in a reasonably sympathetic group. Those in more rural areas noted additional problems of physical access and their dependence on cars (their own or friends') to reach shops at a distance. Even those on higher incomes mentioned reducing other expenditure to maintain their food budget, but people on lower incomes clearly had little room for manoeuvre; many were already budgeting very carefully with little other expenditure they could reduce to buy food.

There was considerable discussion of the trade-off people had to make between price and quality: although certain foodstuffs might be cheap, they were seen as low in healthiness, taste and other elements of quality, and to represent poor value for money. Some referred to widespread availability of particular very cheap commodities (examples given were alcohol and chicken) acting as 'loss leaders' to draw shoppers into supermarkets where value for money was not guaranteed, and parents often regretted the widespread advertising for unhealthy food which added to difficulties of giving their children healthy foods. Many argued that if incomes were to fall further, people would eat even more cheap, unhealthy and lower quality food. In each workshop, there were a few participants who grew some food, partly as a way of saving money, partly for enjoyment and trust in the provenance. Indeed, workshop discussions revealed that while price was an inevitable priority for most, it was not to the exclusion of other considerations, in particular food quality in terms of health and nutrition.

Own household food security?

In the online survey, respondents were invited to respond to Defra's definition of food security in terms of their own experiences of being able to obtain enough affordable, safe and nutritious food to adequately feed their households during the previous 2 years. Only 55% of respondents said they felt able to feed their household adequately all the time (47% of low income vs 70% higher income respondents), and almost a third of those in low-income households or with children said the cost of food was becoming a serious source of stress; almost half the low-income householders found it difficult to afford the variety of food they wanted. A fifth felt that finding affordable food within easy reach of their home was an increasing problem (31% of low income); car ownership only marginally improved the perceived availability of affordable food. There was considerable variation in respondents' confidence in their future household food security, although many thought their food purchasing strategies would soon change, with about half thinking they would spend a higher proportion of income on food, and would be buying different foods to cope with consistent higher food prices (Figure 2).

Why the increase in food prices?

People were asked in both survey and workshops their opinions on why food prices had risen. In the survey, about half the respondents considered they had a good understanding of why, particularly older shoppers, but only a fifth specified reasons when invited to add them. The written responses mainly referred to increased prices for oil/fuel and related costs of transport, or the 'global economic recession': 'The economic crisis which has been fuelled by the credit based financial society that we were encouraged to live in' (survey respondent), along with mention of 'greed' (applied to supermarkets, politicians, bankers, businessmen) and financial specula-tion. Similar comments emerged in more nuanced form in the workshops, where supermarket need for shareholder profit was often cited as cause of rising prices in response to system cost increases. Reductions in food production due to climate

How likely is each of the following to happen?	Extremely unlikely to happen	Using a scale of 1 to 5			Extremely likely to happen	
	1	2	3	4	5	DK/na
	%	%	%	%	%	%
I will be buying different types / cuts of meat to save money	10	10	21	27	21	11
Meat will be an expensive luxury item which I will only buy for special occasions	14	21	22	21	12	11
My household will be eating less variety of food	17	24	25	19	10	5
Food will take up a significantly greater share of my household expenditure	4	9	28	33	21	4

Base: all respondents (1014)

Figure 2. Survey responses: thinking about future food purchasing.

change and drought received rather less mention, although some were aware of increased costs throughout the food system (production, wages, livestock feed) and the impact of biofuel production. A few survey respondents outlined reasons which mirror official reports:

> In the UK, the weakness of the £ against the euro. Worldwide, and also UK: rise in oil prices, growing affluence of middle classes in, e.g. China and India, some poor harvests. (survey respondent)

A small proportion of survey respondents and many workshop participants thought 'the government' was behind increased food prices, sometimes through policies such as cutting subsidies or the Common Agricultural Policy and sometimes because of unresolved issues around food imports versus UK self sufficiency, even though people also recognised that government had, in practice, little control over food prices. Nevertheless, when asked specifically about who should be responsible for food affordability, 80% of survey respondents and the majority of workshop participants thought this primarily lay with government, who they saw as needing to ensure people have access to a wide choice of affordable nutritious food at all times.

Perceptions of 'food security' and responsibility

The actual term 'food security' had very little resonance with the majority of research participants; few workshop participants and only 30% of online respondents recollected having heard the term or contributed a definition when invited to do so. The majority of those who did, and most workshop participants, associated the term 'food security' with food safety, hygiene standards and quality control: 'where food is safe to eat' was a very common response. 'Food safety' itself meant a wide range of things to different people: not genetically modified or irradiated; containing few chemicals or pesticides; not too much salt or calories; free from bacteria or contamination. That food was clearly and trustworthily labelled and tamper-proofed was also often mentioned. Nevertheless, some participants in both research phases conceptualised 'food security' in terms other than as 'food safety'. For example, nearly 20% of survey respondents who gave an answer conceived of it as ensuring sufficient supply to feed global or national populations, and about 6% mentioned household food access. When presented with Defra's definition of food security (see above) of 'availability, accessibility, affordability', workshop participants seemed comfortable with the ideas and were well able to discuss food accessibility and affordability in relation to their households and practices. Food availability was usually seen in terms of what was present in shops, rather than as matters of supply and production, which had little resonance for most participants beyond the debate on biofuels. More detailed exploration of views is in Kneafsey et al. (forthcoming).

During the workshops, people were asked to locate responsibility for ensuring 'food security' through a simple ranking exercise; every time, and despite considerable discussion, the majority saw 'government' as having most responsibility for ensuring food security. This was particularly the case for 'access' and 'affordability for all', although a few higher income participants thought responsibility for the latter lay with 'people and communities' (that is, people should be able to manage their own household budgets). The complexity of the issues was acknowledged and limits to what government could actually do were recognised, given private sector centrality in growing, processing, trading and retailing food. Retailers were seen as having some responsibility for ensuring the affordability of food, though, as mentioned, there was a degree of cynicism as to retailers' motivations and potential commitment to such a public good as 'food security'. Participants were keen on farmers and producers having responsibility for ensuring the availability and quality of food, but none made the connection with government roles in regulating production standards, animal welfare or food safety. Few ranked 'people and communities' as having responsibility, though some felt consumers could be playing a more active role; the main feeling expressed was of consistent side-lining in terms of power and responsibility, with consumers in fact having very little voice or capacity to effect change.

The attribution of roles and responsibilities within the food system were fairly consistent across different workshops, and thus across all income groups (apart from the exception mentioned) and Defra environmental segmentation groups.

Discussion and conclusions

One key mechanism by which current problems in the food system has been indicated is price: the UK general trend in food prices is upwards, despite the fluctuations described earlier, which marks an end to decades of falling food costs, generally rising incomes and a decreasing proportion of income spent on food even by the lowest income quintile. In the economic climate of 2009–2010, as all these trends reversed, 'food security', at national if not household level, re-emerged in policy language if not popular discourse. Of course, food is essentially a private consumption good, public provision in institutions such as schools or hospitals notwithstanding, and notions of 'consumer choice' underpin contemporary UK policy in both public health and food. Thus, engagement with ordinary people to enable their thinking and desires in relation to policy to be taken into account is critical to successful implementation. The research presented here was initiated by the UK Government Department charged with food policy and security (Defra) to discover how people were reacting to increasing food prices and ideas about food security; strikingly, although the work was not structured in these terms, in both the quantitative and qualitative phases, notions of 'health' were widely used as a frame to discuss food, food prices and food security. Many respondents in the quantitative phase, and almost all in the qualitative phase, acknowledged the difficulties increasing food prices were placing on their family budgets; they could clearly articulate consequent changes in behavioural practices and were anxious about likely outcomes for health and well-being. For some, food stress and elements of real food insecurity were already being experienced, especially by those on low incomes, and several expressed considerable uncertainties as to how they would manage in the future as resources got tighter still. The implications for health and well-being (Tarasuk 2001) through not having enough money for appropriate food were clearly recognised by people themselves.

By contrast, while people were well aware of increased food prices and could discuss reasons quite cogently, few were familiar with the term 'food security', despite its policy and increasing media salience. When pressed, many initially discussed it in terms of 'safety' and 'labelling'; this is not as surprising as it might at first seem. 'Safety' is a legitimate meaning of 'security' in other contexts and the safety of food – that it not be contaminated and be conducive to health – has been a clear consumer concern in the UK as elsewhere in Europe for some time (see Lang *et al.* (2009), Morgan *et al.* (2006) and Kjaernes *et al.* (2007), among many). Further, 'labelling' makes sense from a consumer perspective: most people purchase most of their food, usually from supermarkets, interrogating labels to a greater or lesser extent, and labels are thus key to 'food security' where this is taken to mean the consistency, safety and reliability of food being purchased. Despite people's suspicions, usually voiced unprompted, about how reliable labelling actually was, their sense of food security clearly came from knowing food was genuine (it was what it claimed to be) and from label legitimacy (that labels were accurate and trustworthy). In addition, most workshop participants showed good understanding of supermarket strategies in terms of stocking, presentation and pricing, and, in workshops where there were participants with relevant professional experience such as catering or farming, quite sophisticated discussion of problems and policies in relation to wider issues of availability and food supply as well as access were generated.

Once presented with Defra's definition of 'food security' in terms of availability, access and affordability for all, most of those surveyed or in the workshops engaged with the component ideas fairly vigorously and some groups could demonstrate grasp of the complexities. There was little evidence that respondents were unaware of problems facing the food system, particularly as experienced through rising food prices, or that they were not able to understand the component parts. Rather, it is that people are simply not familiar with the terminology 'food security'. Indeed, when subsequently asked towards the end of the online survey whether they themselves experienced food security and in the workshops the extent to which the UK enjoys a state of food security, drawing the Defra definition in both instances, most were clear that 'full food security' had not been achieved, particularly the element of affordability for all.

The issue of responsibility was also critical: there was strong support for government oversight and leadership for all elements of 'food security', particularly over 'access' and 'affordability'. Despite some scepticism that it had capacity, willingness or power to take on the role, the majority of respondents in both phases saw it as government responsibility to ensure that basic food needed for health was affordable for all, with many in the workshops calling for government to intervene in supermarket pricing and profit. That government should be 'in charge' of food circumstances makes sense of people finding it hard to imagine a future where the food system could be very different – even that prices would continue to rise, let alone that some commodities become unaffordable or unobtainable. Government is seen in this way because of its practical responsibility for national and local retail and food distribution infrastructure and its moral responsibility for ensuring that the whole population has physical and economic access to food for health.

To the extent that the market remains the means of delivering nutritional health, people will perforce continue to position themselves as 'economic consumers' – people who have to buy food at the price they can find in local shops; they thus partially locate responsibility for achieving nutritional security with those who have the power to influence food prices (as well as incomes, outside the focus of this research). While many recognised supermarkets' role in setting food prices, they looked to government to exert moral authority over supermarkets, who were seen to be driven by the profit motive rather than care for consumers. Furthermore, considerable research, beyond the scope of this study but to which some of the authors have contributed (Kneafsey *et al.* 2008, Dowler *et al.* 2010), suggests people increasingly seek to express different relationships to food, producers and the food system beyond the merely economic. Choosing food is both a daily act, embedded in unconscious practice, and a longer term more deliberative process, which contributes to expression of identity, culture and care, and is clearly relational in terms of practice and thinking (Beardsworth and Keil 1997, Kjaernes *et al.* 2007, Kneafsey *et al.* 2008). Nevertheless, while those in this study, as elsewhere, see 'health' in wider terms than absence of disease, and food as contributor to health being that which is nourishing, contributing to happiness and general well-being (rather than the correct balance of nutrients and components), they also saw sufficiency of income as key to enabling full expression of food security. This was true even for those committed to own production and creative sourcing through allotments, vegetable box schemes and the like. Public health policy in the UK is exploring new ways to engage with consumers, including interventions in the 'choice architecture' which directs behaviours towards healthier options, otherwise known as 'nudging' (Rayner 2011). Effectiveness of such population-level activities is under debate (Marteau *et al.* 2011) and a recent House of Lords Science and Technology Committee Report (2011) concluded that the evidence supports a range of interventions, including regulation, as necessary to bring about behavioural change. Clearly, the capacity of 'nudge' approaches to ensure the affordability of healthy food is also extremely questionable. Food security at individual and household level cannot be left to the market and state welfare (Dowler 2002, Lang *et al.* 2009); furthermore, mechanisms have to be found which ensure the voices of those living in food insecurity are heard, not least in challenging notions that 'food and nutrition security' can be achieved by informed consumer choice alone.

Acknowledgements

This research was funded by the UK Department of Environment, Food and Rural Affairs, FO04014, Consumer insight into food prices and food security, and the authors are grateful for the permission to publish. They remain entirely responsible for the text and opinions expressed. They are also grateful to those who took part in the online survey and workshops.

Note

1. All differences cited are statistically significant to at least the 5% level (i.e. $p = <0.05$), 95% confidence limits ±2% to 3%.

References

Ambler-Edwards, *et al.*, 2009. *Food futures: rethinking UK strategy*. London: Chatham House.
Beardsworth, A. and Keil, T., 1997. *Sociology on the menu: an invitation to the study of food and society*. London: Routledge.
Braunsberger, K., Wybenga, H., and Gates, R., 2007. A comparison of reliability between telephone and web-based surveys. *Journal of Business Research*, 60, 758–764.

de Schutter, O., 2010. Food commodities speculation and food price crises: regulation to reduce the risks of price volatility. Briefing Note 02. Available from: http://www.iaahp.net/uploads/media/20102309_briefing_note_02_en.pdf [Accessed 24 September 2010].

Defra, 2006. *Food security and the UK: an evidence and analysis paper*. London: Defra. Available from: https://statistics.defra.gov.uk/esg/reports/foodsecurity/foodsecurity.pdf [Accessed 3 September 2009].

Defra, 2008. *A framework for pro-environmental behaviours*. Report January 2008. Available from: http://www.defra.gov.uk/evidence/social/behaviour/documents/behaviours-jan08-report.pdf [Accessed 20 August 2009].

Defra, 2010. *Food statistics pocketbook 2010*. Available from: http://www.defra.gov.uk/evidence/statistics/foodfarm/food/pocketstats/documents/foodpocketbook2010.pdf [Accessed 18 February 2011].

Department of Health, 2010. *Change4Life one year on*. London: Department of Health. Available from: http://www.dh.gov.uk/en/Publicationsandstatistics/Publications/PublicationsPolicyAndGuidance/DH_112529 [Accessed 20 February 2011].

Dowler, E., 2002. Food and poverty in Britain: rights and responsibilities. *Social Policy and Administration*, 36, 698–717.

Dowler, E., 2010. Income needed to achieve a minimum standard of living. *British Medical Journal*, 341, 4070.

Dowler, E., Caraher, M., and Lincoln, P., 2007. Inequalities in food and nutrition: challenging 'lifestyles'. *In*: E. Dowler and N. Spencer, eds. *Challenging health inequalities: from Acheson to 'Choosing Health'*. Bristol: Policy Press, 127–156.

Dowler, E., *et al.*, 2010. 'Doing food differently': reconnecting biological and social relationships through care for food. *In*: N. Charles and R. Carter, eds. *Nature, society and environmental crisis. Sociological review monograph*. Chichester: Wiley-Blackwell, 200–221.

Evans, A., 2008. *Rising food prices: drivers and implications for development*. London: Chatham House.

FAO, 1996. Rome declaration on world food security and world food summit plan of action. *World Food Summit*, 13–17 November 1996. Rome: FAO.

FAO, 2009. *The state of food insecurity in the world 2009: economic crises – impacts and lessons learned*. Rome: Food and Agriculture Organization. Available from: http://www.fao.org/publications/sofi/en/[Accessed 24 September 2010].

Foresight, 2011. *The future of food and farming. Final project report*. London: The Government Office for Science. Available from: http://www.bis.gov.uk/assets/bispartners/foresight/docs/food-and-farming/11-546-future-of-food-and-farming-report.pdf [Accessed 18 February 2010].

Global Food Markets Group (across Whitehall), undated. *The 2007/08 agricultural price spikes: causes and policy implications*. Available from: http://www.defra.gov.uk/foodfarm/food/pdf/ag-price100105.pdf [Accessed 18 February 2011].

Godfray, H.C.J., *et al.*, 2010. Food security: the challenge of feeding 9 billion people. *Science*, 327 (5967), 812–818.

House of Lords Science and Technology Committee, 2011. *Behavioural change*. London: House of Lords Science and Technology Committee Second Report. Available from: http://www.publications.parliament.uk/pa/ld201012/ldselect/ldsctech/179/17902.htm [Accessed 20 July 2011].

HLTF, 2008. *High-level task force on the global food crisis: comprehensive framework for action*. Available from: http://www.who.int/food_crisis/food_crises_july2008.pdf [Accessed 24 September 2010].

IAASTD, 2008. *Agriculture at a crossroads: global summary for decision makers*. Washington: Island Press for the International Assessment of Agricultural Knowledge, Science and Technology for Development (IAASTD). Available from: http://www.islandpress.org/iaastd [Accessed 17 May 2009].

Killeen, D., 2000. Food security: a challenge for Scotland. *In*: J. McCormick, ed. *Healthy food policy: on Scotland's menu?* Edinburgh: Scottish Council Foundation with the Joseph Rowntree Foundation, 17–18.

Kjaernes, U., Harvey, M., and Warde, A., 2007. *Trust in food: a comparative and institutional analysis*. Basingstoke: Palgrave Macmillan.

Kneafsey, M., *et al.*, 2008. *Reconnecting consumers, producers and food: exploring alternatives*. Oxford: Berg.

Kneafsey, M., *et al.*, forthcoming. Consumer perceptions of 'food security' in the United Kingdom. *Journal of Rural Studies*, Special Issue: Food security: Emerging perspectives and responses.

Lang, T., Barling, D., and Caraher, M., 2009. *Food policy: integrating health, environment and society*. Oxford: Oxford University Press.

MacMillan, T. and Dowler, E., 2011. Secure and sustainable? Examining the rhetoric and potential realities of UK food and agriculture policy. *Journal of Agricultural and Environmental Ethics*, online preliminary publication. Available from: http://www.springerlink.com/content/0537k617113tk871/

Marteau, T.M., *et al.*, 2011. Judging nudging: can nudging improve population health? *British Medical Journal*, 342, d228.

Maxwell, S., 1996. Food Security: a post-modern perspective. *Food Policy*, 21 (2), 155–170.

Maxwell, S., 2001. The Evolution of Thinking about Food Security. *In*: S. Devereux and S. Maxwell, eds. *Food Security in Sub-Saharan Africa*. London: ITDG, 13–27.

Maye, D., Holloway, L., and Kneafsey, M., eds, 2007. *Alternative food geographies: representation and place*. London: Elsevier.

Morgan, K., Marsden, T., and Murdoch, J., 2006. *Worlds of food: place, power and provenance in the food chain*. Oxford: Oxford University Press.

Nord, M., *et al.*, 2010. *Household food security in the United States, 2009*. Washington DC: USDA.

ONS, 2010. *Family spending: A report on the 2009 Living Costs and Food Survey*. London: Office for National Statistics.

Patel, R., 2007. *Stuffed and starved: markets, power and the hidden battle for the world food system*. London: Portobello Books.

Patel, R., 2009. What does food sovereignty look like? *Journal of Peasant Studies*, 36 (3), 663–673.

Rayner, M. 2011. Nudge public health: the new laissez-faire? *Food Ethics*, 6, 4, 7–8. Available from: http://www.foodethicscouncil.org/node/622 [Accessed 13 March 2011].

Roberts, P., 2008. *The end of food: the coming crisis in the world food industry*. London: Bloomsbury.

Robertson, A., *et al.*, 2004. *Food and health in Europe: a new basis for action*. Copenhagen: World Health Organisation Regional Office for Europe, WHO Regional Publications, European Series No. 96.

Shaw, D.J., 2007. *World food security: a history since 1945*. Basingstoke: Palgrave Macmillan.

Tarasuk, V.S., 2001. Household food insecurity with hunger is associated with women's food intakes, health and household circumstances. *Journal of Nutrition*, 131, 2670–2676.

The Strategy Unit, 2008. *Food matters: towards a strategy for the 21st century*. London: Cabinet Office.

von Braun, J., (2008). *Food and financial crises: implications for agriculture and the poor*. Washington IFPRI. Available from: http://www.ifpri.org/publication/food-and-financial-crises [Accessed 18 February 2011].

Hunger and nutritional poverty in Germany: quantitative and qualitative empirical insights

Sabine Pfeiffer[a], Tobias Ritter[a] and Andreas Hirseland[b]

[a]Institut für Sozialwissenschaftliche Forschung e.V. (ISF München), Munich, Germany;
[b]Institut für Arbeitsmarkt- und Berufsforschung, Nuremberg, Germany

Despite increasing social inequality, hunger and nutritional poverty are not regarded as phenomena of German reality; Germany's debate on eating patterns is largely dominated by the issue of obesity. The article challenges this view and shows by means of empirical approaches that hunger and nutritional poverty tend to be underestimated in a supposedly affluent society. Due to a lack of appropriate food research in Germany, our study gives quantitative evidence drawn from a combination of studies to show that there is nutritional poverty in Germany, and that social welfare recipients are widely excluded from eating out, arguably an essential form of social and cultural participation. Furthermore, we provide insights, based on a qualitative longitudinal study, into day-to-day coping practices in response to food shortage. As the empirical results show, physiological hunger and hunger for social inclusion by eating out are a reality in contemporary German society. The predominant responses of the German political and social welfare system, however, can be characterised by delegation and denial of the problem and by a tendency to stigmatise the poor.

Poverty, food and eating in Germany

The debate on eating patterns in Europe and especially in the case of Germany appears to be dominated by obesity. According to the German food survey (Nationale Verzehrsstudie – NVS), which was carried out in the 1980s (NVS I) and repeated between 2005 and 2007 (NVS II), one in five people is classified as obese. Most notably, the incidence of excess weight is unequally distributed along the social scale: the higher the level of educational qualifications and per capita income, the lower the body mass index (BMI), and vice versa (Max-Rubner-Institut 2008a, b).

Challenging the dominance of obesity in the debate on eating patterns, we first argue that there is strong empirical evidence that hunger and nutritional poverty exist in the heart of Germany. Although not currently a widespread problem, it is on the increase, but remains largely overlooked and neglected in public and scientific debates. Due to a lack of appropriate and systematic data, we will base our argument on circumstantial evidence from a variety of quantitative data sources.

Furthermore, we argue that this evidence not only gives rise to concerns over social distributive justice and nutritional physiology but also raises complex questions of participation. In modern societies, hunger and nutritional poverty is more than ever both a question of insufficient food rations and a societal and cultural question. Even though we possess 'impressive nutritional versatility' (Beardsworth and Keil 1997, p. 50), food always becomes loaded with meaning as soon as culture and society are involved and is turned into a sign related to each culture's symbolic order. Using the example of eating out, we demonstrate how people in need are systematically excluded from this basic method of participation in contemporary society. Again, we provide circumstantial evidence from different quantitative surveys to emphasise our argument.

Third, we will complement the quantitative overview with a typology of everyday practices of coping with food shortage. This is based on our current qualitative longitudinal study conducted with welfare recipients, which has been running since 2007. Finally, we will briefly look at how the political and societal strategies of dealing with the issue – such as delegation, denial and stigmatisation – might aggravate hunger, nutritional poverty and related problems in Germany.

Quantitative indications of hunger and nutritional poverty in Germany

Hunger could be regarded as the physical expression of too little nourishment (Anderson 1990, p. 1589). According to Feichtinger (1995, p. 295 ff) we can distinguish two types of nutritional poverty; in the case of the material type, food intake does not cover nutritional needs in terms of both quantity and quality. Social nutritional poverty is a barrier to compliance with socially accepted customs and traditions regarding food intake. Although the German food survey (NVS) 2005–2007 provides information on the eating habits and the nutritional status of approximately 20,000 people, it reveals little of the extent of nutritional poverty and hunger in Germany. Whereas systematic and more regular surveys on nutrition in Great Britain[1] or the USA[2] take into consideration poorer population strata or even over-represent them, the German NVS deliberately excluded population groups at a higher risk of nutritional poverty from the study. Therefore, migrants, residents in institutions, persons without a permanent home, children under the age of 14, families with children and elderly people living on their own are clearly under-represented. As this criticism of the NVS I (Kaiser 2001, pp. 44–45) went unheeded in the NVS II (Pfeiffer 2010), we look at other empirical evidence to discuss whether there is hunger and nutritional poverty in Germany.

- *Circumstantial evidence I: Many people are likely to be short of money to spend on food.* According to SOEP[3] 2007, 1% of its respondents have a budget of less than 99 Euros for their total household expenses (i.e. for both food and non-food items) and 7% have a budget of between 100 and 199 Euros. Even from a conservative point of view it can be assumed that the 800,000 people in the group whose household expenditure is under 99 Euros are likely to live in nutritional poverty and experience hunger at least from time to time. This may also hold true for some of the 7% of the population – more than 5 million people – on the budget of between 100 and 199 Euros and thus are presumably suffering from nutritional poverty.[4] Since many households with low household expenditure are on social benefits, a glance at the spending that is possible under the actual welfare conditions of SGB II[5] is telling. The buying power of this benefit is markedly lower compared with welfare benefits before 2005, and is therefore still under judicial and public criticism. Taking into account the inflation rates since 1998 and the VAT increase in 2007, the unemployment benefit entitlement of 351 Euros, valid up to 2009, had a real purchasing power of only 291 Euros (Jaquemoth 2007, pp. 75–80) and its increase to 359 Euros in July 2009 has not substantially changed this situation. Of the standard benefits for single people in 2007, 135 Euros were nominally intended for food and non-alcoholic beverages – a nominal value of 4.5 Euros a day. By way of comparison, the average monthly spending rate on food in one-person households in the old federal states in the year 2000 amounted to over 221 Euros (Hünecke et al. 2004, p. 20 ff) – a daily expenditure of 7.4 Euros. Thus, the amount of money allotted to food spending by the German welfare system today is 40% less than the average expenditure of the population in 2000 – even without factoring in the inflation rate. Thus, welfare recipients rank food in the top two most significant and painful limitations, second only to holidays (Ames 2007) while simultaneously trying to cut back on food as little as possible, especially those in families with children (Wüstendörfer 2008). According to the data of the PASS[6] (2006/2007), almost all welfare recipients go without a daily hot meal for financial reasons (Bernhard 2008, p. 8).

- *Circumstantial evidence II: Germany has experienced a large increase in food banks.* For many people, food banks have become an essential source of nutrition. Currently, 880 food banks support more than one million people with food donations (Federal Association of German Food Banks, press release of 25 May 2011); it is estimated that about half take donations on a regular basis (Normann 2003, p. 143). This is a significant expansion in numbers; in 2005, there were 540 food banks in Germany, compared with just 270 in 2000 (Selke 2009a). In 2001, 75% of the regular food bank customers in Germany were supported by the welfare system; others were homeless or retired (Normann 2003).

Given this circumstantial evidence, it is hardly surprising that the German Society for Nutrition has concluded that eating according to the rules of an optimal mixed diet – currently regarded as the most healthy – is not only difficult to achieve but impossible for welfare recipients above the age of three (Kersting and Clausen 2007). Against this background, the following observation on hunger in Germany is of little reassurance: 'For most poor people, genuine phases of hunger only occur periodically when their housekeeping money runs low' (Barlösius et al. 1995, p. 20).[7] It is in the nature of housekeeping money to periodically run low at the end of the month, meaning 12 times a year. By the beginning of the 1990s, the German social welfare allowance for food was already only sufficient for an average of 19.5 days a month (Roth 1992, p. 8). For the rest of the month, food intake is limited to extremely dull and repetitive meals (Lehmkühler and Leonhäuser 1998); people on social welfare then live on noodles with instant sauces or toast with margarine and jam (Kamensky 2004). In extreme cases, this can add up to 120 days a year, in which those affected conclusively suffer from nutritional poverty and certainly also partially from hunger. Social welfare benefits seem not to provide an appropriate economic basis for adequate nutrition for recipients. Up to 70% of welfare recipients save on food bills; for two-thirds, the budget does not cover the costs of a proper diet (Kaiser 2001, pp. 48–52). Despite the overall unsatisfactory database, in the light of these figures and circumstantial evidence, it can be asserted that there are people in our midst experiencing occasional hunger. Perhaps the number of people experiencing this, the length of time, the frequency and the intensity is of lesser importance than the fact that hunger and nutritional poverty occur at all in German society.

Alimentary participation: the case of eating out

Nutritional poverty in modern societies is not only a question of insufficient food rations, but a societal one. What role do nutrition and food play in our society, i.e. in its social relations, practices and discourses? And which opportunities of social participation are connected with it? Eating is a deep social act and even the most basic and most common decision is a social one, namely, is something edible or not (Beardsworth and Keil 1997, p. 50)? Thus food forms an ineluctable bond between culture and nature.

On this basis, food is credited with playing an important role for the construction of identity (Beardsworth and Keil 1997, p. 53), the development of the self and of emotions (Lupton 1996) and in the socialisation process (Prahl and Setzwein 1999, pp. 121–125). Therefore, what, where and how we eat and cook, i.e. our patterns of food choice, are deeply rooted in the social sphere (Murcott 1998). In this sense, 'man is what he eats' (Feuerbach 1990, p. 358) and 'societies are the way they eat' (Barlösius 1999, p. 9). Thus, food and nutrition are actually the most basic and central participation mechanisms in every social system. By means of the example of eating out,[8] in the following section we want to empirically approach what could be called *alimentary participation* (Pfeiffer 2010, pp. 97–99). Where, how, with whom and on which occasions we go out to eat; how we dress and what we spend on dining out; which cultural setting we choose; whether we are in command of good table manners and know which food is hip; and whether we are moreover able to follow the permanent changes in table and food trends – all of this determines, reveals and enables our degree of success and of belonging to an individualised and pluralistic society. From this perspective, eating out can be regarded as an increasingly relevant point of culmination of alimentary participation, all the more so since the major increase in eating out in developed industrial countries since the 1980s (Beardsworth and Keil 1997, pp. 115–122, Finkelstein 1998, p. 201, Teuteberg 2003).[9] Therefore, if low income and poverty structurally restrict the variety and frequency of eating out occasions, alimentary participation becomes a question of social inequality and of exclusion. But we see empirical evidence pointing to exclusion from alimentary participation as a widespread phenomenon.[10]

- *Circumstantial evidence I: Spending by unemployed households on gastronomic services are far lower than average.* Money has become an essential condition for social participation. Consequently, eating out primarily hinges on socioeconomic status as low-income earners spend significantly less on dining out than average earners (Beardsworth and Keil 1997, p. 116, Warde and Martens 1998, Kamensky 2004). Therefore, a glance at the financial resources spent on dining out refers to the degree of alimentary participation of people living in poverty in Germany. In the absence of data (e.g. in the Report on Poverty and Wealth or the NVS) an estimation by means of data from the Federal Statistical Office (Destatis 2008) seems a viable solution. In 2005, an average employee household had 2343 Euros a month at its disposal for private consumption, of which 134 Euros were spent on accommodation and restaurant services. The jobless household, however, only spends 37 Euros a month on away-from-home meals, of a total consumption expenditure of 1205 Euros a month.

- *Circumstantial evidence II: For unemployed households eating out is rarely an option.* A detailed look reveals that households living on welfare have significantly less financial resources for eating out than the average employed household. A household of welfare recipients on German standard benefits of 2008, consisting of two adults and two children (one under the age of 14, the other under 7), with 1200 Euros a month for private consumption, has roughly 23 Euros to dedicate to eating out for the whole family a month, according to official calculations. This is virtually nothing considering that in 2008, the average bill for dining out in Germany amounted to 14.50 Euros per person (CHD Experts Deutschland 2008). Further evidence of exclusion from alimentary participation in Germany comes from figures showing that while on average Germans eat out 85 times a year (Millstone and Lang 2008, p. 93), 12% of all households in Germany state that they generally cannot afford to dine out (European Quality of Life Survey 2003). This group includes welfare recipients, 76% of whom go without a single monthly visit to a restaurant (Bernhard 2008).

These figures illustrate a wide discrepancy in alimentary participation in the form of eating out in its social meaning, which also involves trying various offerings and dining with different people in different constellations (Pfeiffer 2010). One cannot but agree with Beardsworth and Keil: 'Dining out is experienced and enjoyed by all except the poorest members of society' (1997, p. 118). What is dramatic about this, however, is that we are not talking about the exclusion from one social activity among many but from a basic and essential mode of participation in contemporary society.

Coping with nutritional scarcity and alimentary exclusion

In 2008, in Germany, more than 7.5 million were living on social welfare, representing about 9.5% of the population (Statistisches Bundesamt 2010). Within this group, the greatest proportion are those of working age between 15 and 65 and their respective families. This group have been subject to the workfare-oriented welfare regime implemented by German Social Code II since 2005. While this regime had aimed to get people into employment rapidly, it soon became evident that half became long-term recipients who had to claim benefits for 2 years or more (Graf 2007). These figures suggest that there are a large number of people who face the described shortcomings in nutrition and (alimentary) participation not only occasionally but as a continuing experience in their daily life. This raises the question of how people practically deal with such a situation.

One initial approach stems from our qualitative research project, 'Poverty dynamics and labour market' which aims to reconstruct the patterns of poverty dynamics and their connections to institutional processes of poverty prevention, alleviation and reduction. The project started in January 2006 and concludes in January 2012.[11] In this qualitative longitudinal study, more than 100 welfare recipients as defined by Social Code II have been repeatedly interviewed over a period of approximately 4 years, using biographical in-depth interviews, with most interviews taking place in their home environment (for more details see Hirseland and Lobato 2010). Each interviewee was supposed to be questioned four times over a period of about 4 years. The first wave of interviews started in January 2007 and the fourth one has been completed. The transcribed material consists of 458 qualitative interviews, of which 80 cases were interviewed over all four waves. One aim of this longitudinal study is to analyse how welfare recipients cope with precarious levels of material and non-material resources.

Not only does our qualitative material support the empirical findings described above – for example, with reference to financial restrictions on expenditures for food and nutrition, to exclusion from alimentary participation and to use of food banks – but it also gives some insights into how people cope with a nutritional situation that is, at least at the end of the month, indeed one of nutritional poverty.

Based on in-depth interpretations of the interviews and case comparisons, we have so far been able to identify a variety of interacting conditions that shape the ways in which the interviewees are coping with this restricted nutritional situation: *'objective' factors* like accessibility of food banks and other infrastructural features of food supply, facilities for food storing and cooking; *'subjective' factors* such as the overall attitude to food and eating, e.g. lifestyle, indulgence or modest eating, eating culture and health awareness, shopping patterns and use of food banks, capabilities of household and money management including cooking skills; *'medical' factors*, e.g. illnesses that require special diets; and finally *factors of 'sociality'*, such as caring for others or being cared for, the range and intensity of family and social networks in general and the respective time structure of eating.

In an additional step of our analysis, we were able to elaborate on how those conditions are entwined with each other. In a dialectical and dynamic form of ongoing biographical transformation and sedimentation, they are both reason and result for individual representations of coping types that we described along three analytical dimensions: nutrition and alimentary experiences; biographical acquisition of eating habits; and overall capabilities referring to food. For that reason, 'the needy' are far from being a homogenous group from the nutritional perspective. Up to this point, by following these analytical steps, we have identified a broad variety of individual coping types. The most characteristic of them can be labelled as:

- *Against the odds.* People coping actively with the situation; pragmatic and not shameful use of food banks; making the best of it.
- *Children first.* Subjective feeling of severe restriction of food supply, but trying hard to provide their own children with good and healthy food.
- *Abandonment of quality.* Coping with financial restrictions for food by lowering quality of food. Quantity and comforting food (such as sweets, fatty foods) even of low quality are preferred to healthier food if the costs are higher.

- *Fatalistic abandonment of quality.* Lowering quality of food as a perceived necessity despite the anticipation of serious risks caused by chronic diseases (e.g. diabetes).
- *Abandonment of quantity.* Coping with financial restrictions for food by lowering the quantity of food. Because of the requirements of special diets, due to ideological or religious reasons or just because of a sustainable lifestyle, this type always prefers quality over quantity.
- *Surfing the ups and downs.* Due to different financial situations during the month, this type changes the nutrition and strategies of food supply: simulating normality in the beginning and spiralling downward to an increasingly restricted nutritional situation over the course of the month.
- *Embracing nutrition for sense and structure.* For this type, activities like cooking, eating, and managing of food supplies provide not only practical solutions for the restricted nutritional situation but sense and time structure, too.
- *Enforcing networks.* In order to maintain the food supply, this type depends on social networks: parents, children and friends are visited not only as a social act but also as a means to improve their nutritional situation.
- *Risky food financing.* Due to insufficient economic resources this type tries explicitly to enhance the food supply even in potentially risky ways such as exploiting their own body (e.g. blood donations) or illegal work.

In further analysis of our qualitative material, we will hopefully be able to further specify these initial types in more detail. For the time being one thing seems to hold true: as long as people have to rely on social benefits, they are very likely to suffer from rigid constraints concerning alimentary participation, even amounting to exclusion. This includes a lack of choice. As eating out in restaurants is limited to one occasion every two or three months or less, choice is often restricted to food banks or invitations by friends and family – under the circumstances in question hardly a demonstration of freedom of choice.

Societal forms of dealing with hunger

So far we have attempted to demonstrate that there are strong indications that hunger and lack of alimentary participation have become part of German society and that their degree is widely underestimated. The latter is not only due to a shortage of scientific research on food poverty and related issues but also a matter of how society and politics perceive the problem, and of the way the problem is dealt with. Thus, with delegation, denial, and stigmatisation we refer to three societal coping strategies, which in our opinion are characteristic of current German society (Pfeiffer 2010).

- *Delegation of food security to volunteers and the private sector.* As shown above, virtually all food bank users receive social benefits. On the one hand, the German welfare system apparently fights poverty in a way that brings forth nutritional poverty, on the other hand, however, food security seems to be no longer regarded as a function of the state. This indicates a retrograde move, for until recently food security used to be a vital source of legitimacy of political rule (Barlösius 1999, p. 9–10, Montanari 1999, pp. 105–106, Gratzer 2005, p. 16 ff). Modern state administration was the first to invent a rational system of feeding the poor, which orients itself on 'economic calculability' and attempts to free itself from the 'odium of poor relief' (Teuteberg 2009, pp. 49–56). Today, by contrast, the state explicitly delegates the task of overcoming nutritional poverty to private economy and voluntary activities. As a result, the food security of people living in poverty is to a great extent left to chance and in some cases it is purely arbitrary. Which foodstuffs are available to them, when, where and in which quantities or qualities, where food banks are founded and are open to the public – all these factors are not the result of political or administrative objectives but highly dependent on decisions by local entrepreneurs and volunteers. Although more and more people in Germany are forced to rely on food banks for their regular nutritional supply, the German welfare state delegates food security to this realm of entrepreneurial and voluntary freedom and therefore beyond the reach of governmental interventions.

- *Legacy of the post-war German 'economic miracle', or the denial of 'which must not be'*. Following Paugam (2008, p. 191), in Germany, the existence of poverty is being 'denied or underestimated' to a greater extent than in the rest of Europe. An important sociocultural reason for this specifically strong denial of poverty seems to be the post-war 'economic miracle' (Butterwegge 2009). What applies to poverty applies all the more to hunger. After all, no other phase in German history is as closely and lastingly linked to an abundance of food as in the 1950s, and in the media, the reconstruction of post-war Germany is more closely linked to images of piles of sausages than to smoking chimneys. Up to now, these images have imprinted the phrase, 'Nobody needs to starve' upon Germany's collective self-perception. Thus, poverty, and especially, hunger have to be negated both in public opinion and in political action. The denial of the one intensifies and entails the denial of the other: if there is no hunger, there cannot be poverty – and vice versa.

- *Physical characteristics and food bank-adequate poverty – new forms of stigmatisation*. New poverty, precarity and new underclass (Castel and Dörre 2009), exclusion (Kronauer 2002, Bauman 2005), social in/justice (Kronauer 2007, Dubet 2008, Becker 2009) and the debate on 'the superfluous' (Bude and Willisch 2007, Bude 2008), the topic of social inequality is currently booming in German sociology. One aspect of increasing social inequality that so far has only been addressed on the sidelines is stigmatisation in connection with nutritional poverty, which occurs in three variants. First, visibly unhealthy eating habits that result in being overweight are stigmatised. The 'crusade against fat people' (Schmidt-Semisch and Schorb 2007) is in full swing – despite doubts about the usefulness of the body mass index (Campos 2004, Spiekermann 2007). Second, the poor have always been suspected of having the wrong lifestyle, self-indulgent and/or inappropriate (Feichtinger 1995, p. 301 ff, Barlösius 1999, p. 63 ff). With a bourgeois wagging finger, the underclass is denied its 'happy meal' (Schorb 2007). Physical characteristics like obesity thus become a signal for exclusion (Bude 2008, p. 106); clandestinely and at the same time, intensified and popularised by the media and its allusions to 'trash', a 'physiognomy of the social classes' is developing (ibid.: p. 110). And third, prospectively and increasingly, a food bank-specific stigmatisation is developing. Food banks are intersecting points, at which the superfluous goods of the affluent society encounter 'the superfluous' members of that society (Selke 2009b, p. 30). Thus, food bank users become subject to stigmatisation, for the use of food banks publicly documents not only the exclusion from alimentary participation but also the potentiality of hunger.

Delegation, denial and stigmatisation of hunger and nutritional poverty in Germany are three ways of dealing with these phenomena that are socially prevalent in German society and government. They are closely interrelated and mutually reinforced each other. If they continue to prevail, they might contribute to an increase in nutritional poverty and hunger. Here, social sciences have a contribution to make towards challenging the orthodoxy. The best way to do so is to orient its methods and concepts to the realisation that alimentary deprivation can also become an existential problem for many people in German society.

Notes

1. National Food Survey (NFS).
2. National Health and Nutrition Examination Survey (NHANES).
3. The German Socio-Economic Panel Study (SOEP) is a wide-ranging representative longitudinal study of private households, see: http://www.diw.de/soep.
4. These figures do not yet include those without households, i.e. the estimated 300,000 homeless people in Germany (Die Zeit, 5.3.2009), and little is known about their diet (Kutsch 1995).
5. The second book of the German Social Code (SGB II) came into effect on 1 January 2005. It combined former unemployment benefit and social welfare to form a uniform basic income support scheme for those capable of work but in need of support (currently, 364 Euros plus housing costs a month). Together with benefits that ensure a basic standard of living, this support scheme also aims at retaining, restoring or improving the employability of those requiring support.
6. The Panel Study 'Labour Market and Social Security' is an annual household survey which is conducted by the Institute for Employment Research (IAB), see: http://fdz.iab.de/en/FDZ_Individual_Data/PASS.aspx.
7. All quotations originally in German have been translated by the authors.
8. In accord with the cited literature and data, we define eating out as eating in restaurants, pubs and take-away facilities of all kinds but not eating in the homes of friends and family.
9. Two mutually reinforcing although seemingly contradictory trends set the increasingly rapid pace of change: the pluralisation of gastronomic choice and the standardisation of gastronomic services (Prahl and Setzwein 1999, pp. 58–61). Despite these changes and although there seems to be a shift from collective to individualistic moral patterns on eating (Barlösius 2004), the motives for going to restaurants have barely changed over the course of time: then and now the point is ultimately the simultaneous satisfaction of physical and social needs (Mennell 2003).
10. Due to the lack of a consistent set of data, the variety of methodological heterogeneous surveys we mention to support our point do not provide an overall standardised cost for their calculations.
11. The project is part of the evaluation of Social Code II by the German Federal Ministry of Labour and Social Affairs (Bundesministerium für Arbeit und Soziales). It is executed by the Institute for Employment Research (Institut für Arbeitsmarkt- und Berufsforschung,

Nuremberg) in collaboration with the Hamburg Institute for Social Research (Hamburger Institut für Sozialforschung; Hamburg) and the Institute for Social Science Research Munich (Institut für Sozialwissenschaftliche Forschung e.V.; Munich).

References

Ames, A., 2007. *Ich Hab's Mir Nicht Ausgesucht. . . . Die Erfahrungen der Betroffenen mit der Umsetzung und den Auswirkungen des SGB II.* Mainz.

Anderson, S.A., 1990. The 1990 Life Sciences Research Office (LSRO) report on nutritional assessment defined terms associated with food access. Core indicators of nutritional state for difficult to sample populations. *Journal of Nutrition*, 102, 1559–1660.

Barlösius, E., 1999. *Soziologie des Essens: Eine Sozial- und kulturwissenschaftliche Einführung in die Ernährungsforschung.* Weinheim, München: Juventa.

Barlösius, E., 2004. Von der Kollektiven zur Individualisierten Essmoral? Über das "Gute Leben" und die widersprüchlichen Grundmuster alltäglichen Essens. *In*: H.-J. Teuteberg, ed. *Die Revolution am Esstisch. Neue Studien zur Nahrungskultur im 19./20. Jahrhundert.* Stuttgart, Germany: Steiner, 39–50.

Barlösius, E., Feichtinger, E., and Köhler, B.M., 1995. Armut und Ernährung – Problemaufriß eines wiederzuentdeckenden Forschungsgebiets. *In*: E. Barlösius, E. Feichtinger, and B.M. Köhler, eds. *Ernährung in der Armut.* Berlin: Edition Sigma, 11–26.

Bauman, Z., 2005. *Verworfenes Leben. Die Ausgegrenzten der Moderne.* Hamburg: Hamburger Edition.

Beardsworth, A. and Keil., T., 1997. *Sociology on the menu: invitation to the study of food and society.* London, New York, NY: Routledge.

Becker, J., 2009. Das Unbehagen in der Gesellschaft. Soziale Ungleichheiten und Ungerechtigkeitserfahrungen in Deutschland. *In*: S. Selke, ed. *Tafeln in Deutschland.* Wiesbaden: VS Verlag für Sozialwissenschaften, 107–135.

Bernhard, C., 2008. Was Fehlt Bei Hartz IV? Zum Lebensstandard der Empfänger von Leistungen nach SGB II. *Informationsdienst Soziale Indikatoren (ISI)*, 40, 7–10.

Bude, H., 2008. *Die Ausgeschlossenen. Das Ende vom Traum einer gerechten Gesellschaft.* München: Hanser.

Bude, H. and Willisch, A., eds., 2007. *Exklusion: Die Debatte über die 'Überflüssigen'.* Frankfurt/M.: Suhrkamp.

Butterwegge, C., 2009. *Armut in einem reichen Land: Wie das Problem verharmlost und verdrängt wird.* Frankfurt/M.: Campus.

Campos, P., 2004. *The obesity myth: why America's obsession with weight is hazardous to your health.* New York, NY: Gotham.

Castel, R. and Dörre, K., 2009. Die Wiederkehr der sozialen Unsicherheit. *In*: R. Castel, and K. Dörre, eds. *Prekarität, Abstieg, Ausgrenzung: Die soziale Frage am Beginn des 21. Jahrhunderts.* Frankfurt/M., New York, NY: Campus, 21–34.

CHD Experts Deutschland, 2008. *Juli 2008 – Gastro-Durchschnittsbon in Europa* [online]. Lyon, France: CHD Experts. Available from: http://www.chd-expert.de/zahl_des_monats.php [Accessed 3 December 2009].

Destatis, 2008. *Datenreport 2008: Der Sozialbericht für Deutschland.* Wiesbaden: Destatis.

Dubet, F., 2008. *Ungerechtigkeiten. Zum subjektiven Ungerechtigkeitsempfinden am Arbeitsplatz.* Hamburg: Hamburger Edition.

Feichtinger, E., 1995. Armut und Ernährung im Wohlstand. Topographie eines problems. *In*: E. Barlösius, E. Feichtinger, and B.M. Köhler, eds. *Ernährung in der Armut.* Berlin: Edition Sigma, 291–305.

Feuerbach, L., 1990. Die Naturwissenschaft und die Revolution. *In*: W. Schuffenhauer and L. Feuerbach, eds. *Gesammelte Werke, Band 10: Kleinere Schriften III. 1846–1850*. Berlin: Akademie, 347–376.

Finkelstein, J., 1998. Dining out: the hyperreality of appetite. *In*: R. Scapp, and B. Seitz, eds. *Eating culture*. New York, NY: State University Press, 201–215.

Graf, T., 2007. *Die Hälfte war zwei Jahre lang durchgehend bedürftig*. Nürnberg: Institut für Arbeitsmarkt- und Berufsforschung, IAB-Kurzbericht 17/2007.

Gratzer, W., 2005. *Terrors of the table: the curious history of nutrition*. Oxford: Oxford University Press.

Hirseland, A. and Lobato, P., 2010. *Armutsdynamik und Arbeitsmarkt. Entstehung, Verfestigung und Überwindung von Hilfebedürftigkeit bei Erwerbsfahigen*. Nürnberg: Institut für Arbeitsmarkt- und Berufsforschung.

Hünecke, K., Fritsche, U.R., and Eberle, U., 2004. *Lebenszykluskosten für Ernährung*. Freiburg: Öko-Institut.

Jaquemoth, M., 2007. Iudex non calculat. Hartz IV auf dem Prüfstand der Haushaltsökonomik. *In*: S. Höflacher, *et al.*, eds. *Oikos (2010) – Haushalte und Familien im Modernisierungsprozess*. Bonn: University Press, 63–100.

Kaiser, C., 2001. *Ernährungsweisen von Familien mit Kindern in Armut*. Stuttgart: Ibidem.

Kamensky, J., 2004. Pizza, Pommes und Probleme – Ernährungsarmut heute. *In*: B. Grzybowski and L. Müller, eds. *Dokumentation des 3. Bremer Forums Gesundheitlicher Verbraucherschutz am 03*. November 2003 in Bremen. Bremen: Senator für Arbeit, Frauen, Gesundheit, Jugend und Soziales, 21–27.

Kersting, M. and Clausen, K., 2007. Wie teuer ist eine gesunde Ernährung für Kinder und Jugendliche? *ErnährungsUmschau*, 9, 508–153.

Kronauer, M., 2002. *Exklusion. Die Gefährdung des Sozialen im hoch entwickelten Kapitalismus*. Frankfurt/M., New York: Campus.

Kronauer, M., 2007. Neue soziale Ungleichheiten und Ungerechtigkeitserfahrungen Herausforderungen für eine Politik des Sozialen. *WSI-Mitteilungen*, 7, 365–372.

Kutsch, T., 1995. Berber-Kost. Ernährungs- und Überlebensmuster der Nicht-Seßhaften. *In*: E. Barlösius, E. Feichtinger, and B.M. Köhler, eds. *Ernährung in der Armut*. Berlin: Edition Sigma, 254–267.

Lehmkühler, S.H. and Leonhäuser, I.-U., 1998. Armut und Ernährung. *Spiegel der Forschung*, 15 (2), 74–82.

Lupton, D., 1996. *Food, the body and the self*. London: Sage.

Max Rubner-Institut, ed., 2008a. *Nationale Verzehrsstudie II – Ergebnisbericht*, Teil 1. Karlsruhe: Bundesforschungsinstitut für Ernährung und Lebensmittel.

Max Rubner-Institut, ed., 2008b. *Nationale Verzehrsstudie II – Ergebnisbericht*. Teil 2. Karlsruhe: Bundesforschungsinstitut für Ernährung und Lebensmittel.

Mennell, S., 2003. Eating in the public sphere in the nineteenth and twentieth centuries. *In*: M. Jacobs, and P. Scholliers, eds. *Eating out in Europe: picnics, gourmet dining and snacks since the late eighteenth century*. Oxford: Berg, 245–260.

Millstone, E. and Lang, T., 2008. *The atlas of food: who eats what, where, and why*. London: Earthscan.

Montanari, M., 1999. *Der Hunger und der Überfluß*. München: C.H.Beck.

Murcott, A., 1998. Food choice, the social sciences and "the nation's diet" research programme. Introduction. *In*: A. Murcott, ed. *The nation's diet: the social science of food choice*. London: Longman, 1–22.

Normann, K.V., 2003. *Evolution der Deutschen Tafeln*. Bad Neuenahr: Wehle.

Paugam, S., 2008. *Die elementaren Formen der Armut*. Hamburg: Hamburger Edition.

Pfeiffer, S., 2010. Hunger in der Überflussgesellschaft. *In*: S. Selke, ed. *Tafeln in Deutschland*. Wiesbaden: VS Verlag für Sozialwissenschaften, 91–107.

Prahl, H.-W. and Setzwein, M., 1999. *Soziologie der Ernährung*. Wiesbaden: VS Verlag für Sozialwissenschaften.

Roth, R., 1992. *Über den Monat am Ende des Geldes*. Frankfurt/M.: DVS.

Schmidt-Semisch, H. and F. Schorb, eds., 2007. *Kreuzzug gegen Fette: Sozialwissenschaftliche Aspekte des gesellschaftlichen Umgangs mit Übergewicht und Adipositas*. Wiesbaden: VS Verlag für Sozialwissenschaften.

Schorb, F., 2007. Keine 'Happy Meals' für die Unterschicht! Zur symbolischen Bekämpfung der Armut. *In*: H. Schmidt-Semisch, and F. Schorb, eds. *Kreuzzug gegen Fette*. Wiesbaden: VS Verlag für Sozialwissenschaften, 107–124.

Selke, S., ed., 2009a. *Tafeln in Deutschland: Aspekte einer Sozialen Bewegung zwischen Nahrungsmittelumverteilung und Armutsintervention*. Wiesbaden: VS Verlag für Sozialwissenschaften.

Selke, S., ed., 2009b. Tafeln und Gesellschaft. Soziologische Analyse eines polymorphen Phänomens. *In*: S. Selke, ed. *Tafeln in Deutschland*. Wiesbaden: VS Verlag für Sozialwissenschaften, 9–38.

Spiekermann, U., 2007. Übergewicht und Körperdeutungen im 20. Jahrhundert. *In*: H. Schmidt-Semisch, and F. Schorb, eds. *Kreuzzug gegen Fette*. Wiesbaden: VS Verlag für Sozialwissenschaften, 35–56.

Statistisches Bundesamt, 2010. *Soziale Mindestsicherung in Deutschland 2008*. Wiesbaden: Statistisches Bundesamt.

Teuteberg, H.J., 2003. The rising popularity of dining out in German restaurants in the aftermath of modern urbanization. *In*: M. Jacobs, and P. Scholliers, eds. *Eating out in Europe*. Oxford: Berg, 281–299.

Teuteberg, H.J., 2009. Historische Vorläufer der Lebensmitteltafeln in Deutschland. *In*: S. Selke, ed. *Tafeln in Deutschland: Aspekte einer Sozialen Bewegung zwischen Nahrungsmittelumverteilung und Armutsintervention*. Wiesbaden: VS Verlag für Sozialwissenschaften, 41–63.

Warde, A. and Martens., L., 1998. A sociological approach to food choice: the case of eating out. *In*: A. Murcott, ed. *The nation's diet*. London: Longman, 129–144.

Wüstendörfer, W., 2008. *Dass man immer nein sagen muss Eine Befragung der Eltern von Grundschulkindern mit Nürnberg-Pass*. Nürnberg: Amt für Existenzsicherung und Soziale Integration.

'It's a full time job being poor': understanding barriers to diabetes prevention in immigrant communities in the USA

Claudia Chaufan[a], Sophia Constantino[b] and Meagan Davis[b]

[a]Department of Social and Behavioral Sciences, Institute for Health and Aging, School of Nursing, University of California San Francisco, 3333 California Street, San Francisco, CA 94118, USA; [b]Institute for Health and Aging, University of California San Francisco, 3333 California Street, San Francisco, CA 94118, USA

This study explores the social determinants of diabetes in a low-income, Latino, and immigrant neighborhood in a Californian city, emphasizing food environments. We conducted focus groups and semi-structured interviews of a convenience sample of staff and clients at a local non-governmental organization. Eight themes emerged as key barriers to healthy eating: (1) cost of food *vis-à-vis* income; (2) transportation; (3) language; (4) stigma; (5) immigration status; (6) insufficient formal/informal food assistance; (7) work conditions; and (8) competing basic needs/constraints of poverty. We conclude that the public health and health education rhetoric of 'individual choice' is a barrier in itself to understanding the diabetes epidemic, and that without the recognition and understanding of, and intervention upon, socioeconomic, policy, and political barriers to healthy lifestyles, the prevention of diabetes will remain out of reach.

Introduction

The increase in rates of type 2 diabetes (hereafter diabetes) over the past three decades has been labeled a pandemic; addressing this pandemic is considered a health and economic imperative (The Lancet 2011). Major reports and articles on diabetes have underscored that unhealthy lifestyles, largely poor diets and physical inactivity, play a critical role in the incidence and prevalence of diabetes, and have called for redoubling efforts to raise awareness about the disease, improve diagnostic tools, or educate the population on personal preventive strategies (Department of Health and Human Services (DHHS) 2003, Zimmet 2003, Naser *et al.* 2006, UnitedHealth Center for Health Reform & Modernization 2010). In contrast, far less emphasis has been placed on the well-established social determinants influencing those lifestyles and on the public policies responsible for those determinants, even as the World Health Organization (WHO) Commission for the Social Determinants of Health has deemed these determinants responsible for the greatest global burden of disease

(Commission on Social Determinants of Health (CSDH) 2008). Understanding how these social determinants affect the distribution of diabetes and preventive efforts is critical to rein on the pandemic.

In this article, we explore socioeconomic barriers to healthy lifestyles, with a special emphasis on barriers to healthy eating, in a low-income Latino immigrant neighborhood in Northern California. While our study is empirical, its goal is primarily conceptual: to draw on our data in order to illustrate the sociopolitical context of the social determinants of health (SDH) in general and of diabetes in particular. An ancillary goal is to propose that a social justice perspective, which calls for an equitable distribution of health-relevant social resources, must be integral to any intervention that purports to tackle diabetes and comparable chronic diseases.

Poverty and basic human needs in the USA

As poverty rates in the USA continue to rise, families increasingly struggle to meet basic needs such as housing, health care, and food. As the latest US Census Bureau report revealed, the number of people living in poverty in 2010 rose for a third consecutive year, reaching a record high of 15.1% – 46.2 million, or one in six Americans, the highest number since the US Census Bureau began tracking such data more than 50 years ago. The report also showed that children under 18 suffer the highest poverty rate, with one in five children living in poverty, and one in ten living in deep poverty, defined as an income of $11,000 for a family of four (compared to the poverty threshold for a family of four, of $22,314 for that same year). Importantly, the report also revealed that Hispanics and blacks together accounted for 54% of the poor, with whites at 9.9% and Asians at 12.1% (US Department of Commerce Economics and Statistics Administration US Census Bureau 2011).

As poverty has increased, so has the gap between the richest and poorest segments of American society. Between the late 1980s and the late 1990s, in most states the income gap between the top 20% of families and the bottom 20% of families grew, whereas the income gap between high- and low-income families increased in all but four states, and the gap between the average incomes of middle-income families and of the richest 20% of families expanded in all but six (Bernstein *et al.* 2000). At the same time, average household income has experienced a steady decline (Irons 2007), and wages have barely moved, even as workers' productivity has risen (Baker 2007).

Similarly, access to affordable housing, defined as one that consumes no more than 30% of household income (whether in rent or mortgage), is increasingly limited: according to the Department of Housing and Urban Development, an estimated 12 million renter and homeowner households now pay more than 50% of their annual incomes for housing (US Department of Housing and Urban Development). This means that a full-time worker supporting a family of four and earning the minimum wage cannot afford the local fair-market rent for a two-bedroom apartment anywhere in the USA (US Department of Housing and Urban Development). The situation is compounded by close to 8 million jobs forever lost since 2007 to the Great Recession, which has also thrust over 8 million households into foreclosure (RealtyTrack – National Real Estate Trends).

As unemployment rates remain high and the size of the labor force drops because discouraged workers stop looking for a job (Baker 2010), in a system strongly dependent on employer-sponsored commercial health coverage, the ranks of the uninsured continue to rise. In 2009, the number of individuals with health insurance had decreased for the first time since this data were collected in 1987, from 255.1 million to 253.6 million, especially in the commercial health insurance sector (partially compensated for by an increase in public programs enrollment, which reached its highest at 30.6%; US Department of Commerce Economics and Statistics Administration US Census Bureau 2010). By 2010, the number of Americans with employer-provided insurance had continued to decline, with the ranks of the uninsured hovering just below 50 million, the highest number in more than two decades (US Department of Commerce Economics and Statistics Administration US Census Bureau 2011).

Finally, and relevant to our study, the number of individuals who rely on food assistance has soared: according to the US Department of Agriculture in August of 2010, 42,389,619 Americans received food stamps, a 17% rise from the same time a year ago, up by 58.5% from August 2007, before the recession began (US Department of Agriculture 2011). This decade-long, dramatic deterioration of the living conditions of millions of American families does not bode well for population health.

Immigrants in the USA

Meeting basic human needs is particularly challenging for immigrant families that suffer multiple forms of discrimination, even as immigrants as a group make important contributions to the US economy and society. These contributions include supplying skilled workers in occupations seen as experiencing labor shortage, or ensuring diversity by increasing the number of individuals from countries historically underrepresented in the US population, both key goals of US immigration policy (Physicians for Human Rights 2000).

Discrimination against immigrants is caused at least in part by a number of myths, for instance, the belief that immigrants do not pay taxes. The reality, however, is that immigrants, documented or not, pay taxes, even more than they receive in benefits. In fact, many immigrants, 74% of whom are incidentally documented, do not seek any form of public assistance, for fear of deportation in the case of the undocumented, or, in the case of documented immigrants, for fear of being perceived as a 'burden to the state' and denied or stripped of citizenship rights (Physicians for Human Rights 2000). Finally, and again against popular belief, immigrants tend to use fewer health services, thus spend less, when compared to American-born individuals – per capita total health care expenditures of immigrants have been estimated 55% lower than those of US-born persons, and expenditures for uninsured and publicly insured immigrants are approximately half those of their US-born counterparts (Mohanty et al. 2005).

Public policy and the SDH inequalities

Deteriorating living conditions take a huge toll on population health, and are an important source of health inequalities. Given the increasingly interconnected nature of contemporary society and the effects of macroeconomic processes on global health, between the years 2005 and 2008, the WHO established the CSDH to gather evidence that could inform public policies addressing those inequalities. The final report drew special attention to the SDH, which the CSDH defined as the 'causes of the causes', or root causes of ill health and health inequalities, meaning the living conditions, together with their social, political, and cultural contexts within which individuals live, work, play, and age (CSDH 2008). The CSDH concluded that the SDH are the strongest determinants of health and of health inequalities, between and within countries. They operate at global, national, and local levels, shaping social norms, interpersonal relationships, institutional arrangements, and the distribution of societal goods and burdens. In order to reduce health inequalities, argued the CSDH, it is critical to look beyond the immediate, i.e., biological and behavioral, causes of disease and reach out to those living conditions such as access to basic sanitation, water, universal primary and secondary education, safe environments that facilitate healthy food choices and physical activity, and employment that provides 'financial security, social status, personal development, social relations and self-esteem, and protection from physical and psychosocial illness' (CSDH 2008). The CSDH also underscored that if health inequalities are to be successfully reduced, it behooves governments and policy makers to address the SDH through compre-hensive and integrated public health, social, and economic policies.

Diabetes and the biology of poverty

Diabetes is one of many diseases importantly influenced by the SDH. It is characterized by insufficient production or uptake of insulin by the tissues, which result in elevated levels of blood glucose. In the USA, close to 25 million individuals 20 years or older, or 11.3% of all people in this age group, live with diabetes, a number that increases to 104 million individuals in this same age group, or 46% of individuals in this group, when cases of pre-diabetes are included (pre-diabetes is a condition in which individuals have elevated levels of blood glucose not high enough to meet the diagnostic criteria of diabetes yet high enough to elevate the risk of heart disease, stroke, or diabetes itself). Diabetes is also a major cause of heart disease and stroke, and the leading cause of kidney disease, new cases of blindness, and non-traumatic limb amputations among adults in the USA. Individuals affected by diabetes are twice as likely to die as those of similar age without the disease (Centers for Disease Control and Prevention (CDC) 2011).

The explosion of diabetes has taken a toll on all social groups, affecting 'the old and the young, men and women, all racial and ethnic groups, the rich and the poor' (Diabetes Research Working Group 1999, p. 15). Nevertheless, diabetes is not an equal opportunity disease, and in the USA as elsewhere it has taken a dispropor-tionate toll on minorities and on the poor, categories that often overlap. After adjusting for population age differences, rates of diabetes among people 20 years of age or more are 7.1% among non-Hispanic whites, 8.4% among Asian Americans, 11.8% among Hispanics (13.3% among Mexican Americans), and 12.6% among non-Hispanic blacks (CDC 2011). In Appalachia, diabetes is increasing at a disturbing speed among the poor, whites and ethnic minorities alike (Wright 2003). Similarly, a Japanese study found that eight times as many low-status workers as high-status workers had diabetes (Morikawa et al. 1997), and a Finnish study found that among diabetic males, almost twice as many blue-collar workers as white-collar workers died in a 5-year period (Forssas *et al.* 2003).

We have labeled this well-established relationship between the SDH and diabetes the 'biology of poverty' (Chaufan 2008). This biology is produced by a combination of mechanisms operating since conception, and which include fetal malnutrition (Barker 2003), poorly controlled diabetes during pregnancy (Jovanovic and Pettitt 2001), stunting in young children (Branca and Ferrari 2002), food insecurity (Seligman *et al.* 2007), and lack of access to timely and quality medical care (White *et al.* 2009), among others. These mechanisms, the product of social exclusion and of an inequitable distribution of resources necessary for health, are also responsible for the intergenerational, social and biological (albeit not genetic) transmission of diabetes (Chaufan 2008).

Despite the evidence causally relating the distribution of diabetes and the SDH, in North America public and private agencies alike typically promote prevention strategies that focus on lifestyle modification, either ignoring or merely paying lip service to how the SDH, especially material deprivation, lead to important differences in the distribution of diabetes in the population (Chaufan 2006, Raphael *et al.* 2011). Thus recognizing and understanding the role of the SDH, and importantly, of the social and economic policies shaping their distribution, is a critical first step to developing effective and sustainable interventions to stem the tide of the diabetes epidemic.

This study

This study was conducted in a city in Northern California, within a neighborhood heavily populated by Latinos. We interviewed a convenience sample of staff serving a low-income community at a local non-governmental organization (NGO) and their Latino immigrant and monolingual clients, most of them Mexican immigrants (two of them from El Salvador). We interviewed all but one staff member ($N = 6$) and conducted two focus groups of a total of 15 clients. Elsewhere, we provide a detailed account of the demographics of our participant population (Chaufan *et al.* 2011). Interviews and focus groups were audio-recorded, translated, and transcribed (when necessary) and thematically analyzed by two of the three investigators (the first author is bilingual) using Atlas Ti, in search for themes illustrating socioeconomic barriers to healthy eating. The study was funded by the School of Nursing at the University of California in San Francisco and approved by the Ethics Review Board at the same institution.

Results

Barriers to healthy eating included the high price of healthy foods (and the comparatively low price of unhealthy foods), inadequate transportation to food outlets, limitations of food assistance, employment, and work conditions, and lastly, competing needs stemming from the sheer constraints of poverty.

In the view of participants, the greatest barrier to healthy eating was the high price of food. As we have documented elsewhere, access to healthy foods in our target neighborhood was importantly impaired by high prices in the local stores, where the price of the Thrifty Food Market Basket was substantially higher than the reference price provided by the US Department of Agriculture, from 14% to as much as 36%, and where between 18% and 26% of the items recommended in the Thrifty Food Plan were missing (Chaufan *et al.* 2011). This barrier was particularly felt among participants who had diabetes or were known to be at higher risk due to their family background. In contrast, 'junk food' was very inexpensive and readily available.

> Researcher: In your opinion, are clients buying [junk food] because of the prices?
> G (staff): Yeah, they are cheaper, and I mean, Mexican stores usually have vegetables around, but they are cheaper if you go to [the chain supermarket]. But I don't think anybody goes and buys their vegetables there, you know. Not ever.
> Y (staff): Who doesn't have a dollar? You can get a Coke, I think, or the Big Gulps at the 7–11. So, I mean, they're cheap. And think of where they put these products-right where it's easily visible and accessible along with *People* magazine and all of that stuff. It's marketing. Teenagers, especially, make those choices. And they market to that.

Clients' views on these matters were very similar:

> GE: If you want good food, it's expensive.
> P: In Mexico, [street] markets ("tiendas") are very popular [...]. During the season, even good quality produce is inexpensive. But [in the USA], even if it's seasonal produce remains expensive.
> D: Well, if you consider our income, it's expensive.
> J: For instance, I am diabetic. I now know I must eat vegetables...and sometimes we don't have enough money to buy that special food for me.
> L: That soup, "Marucha". It's instant. And it's very cheap.
> I: But it has lots of calories, lots of carbohydrates
> M: Another thing, even if you don't have a lot of money there's whole pizza for as little as 4 dollars.

Problems of transportation to food outlets compounded the problem of high prices. Most clients reported having to choose between lower prices and long commutes by public transportation, taking up several hours at a time and carrying multiple bags, or higher prices at closer-by stores, where often they are also forced to shop due to time constraints (e.g., holding multiple low-paying jobs). Additionally, language and stigma considerations mattered to clients' food purchasing practices. For example, none of our participants reported attending the local farmers markets where they can use formal food assistance resources (known as 'food stamps') and buy high quality produce. This is because while the stigma associated with food assistance has largely been eliminated by replacing the old paper stamps with credit-card looking cards, their use is still a problem at these markets because in order to purchase goods, clients must decide *first* how much they will spend, and *then* receive tokens worth a fixed amount (1 dollar) with which they can pay for their food.

> R (staff): [In the market] they do take food stamps. They slide the EBT ('food stamp') card and hand them tokens. But clients have to know how much they will spend [ahead of time]. Researcher: Does that mean that it's more difficult?
> R: Yeah! It's not easy, it's kind of discrimination. Last time I talked to the lady (at the food stamp booth) and she said that people are still confused about how to manage or use their tokens, and they won't come at all.

To note, as customers swipe their card at the EBT stand, they can get as few or as many tokens as they want. The downside, however, is that they do not receive change for amounts in-between whole dollars. So if the total comes to, for instance, $5.50, they must still give 6 tokens, i.e., $6. This means that the system as it stands forces people to either pay more, or purchase more, than they otherwise would, or else their money goes to waste. This is very inconvenient for those on a limited budget, for whom every penny counts.

In addition, most attendants at the market do not speak Spanish. One staff member explained that families would not go to the farmers' market unless they had a bilingual member, often their child, and that one key reason they chose to shop at local food stores, despite higher prices and worse quality, was because they felt 'more comfortable because they speak Spanish'.

We also found that immigration status was a critical barrier to accessing formal food assistance. The enrollment process is lengthy, usually requiring assistance by trained personnel and documentation that many clients do not have. One staff member explained that a 100% of their clients would be eligible if only their income were considered (all but one client participant lived under 100% of the poverty line). However, only 50% actually received food assistance due to barriers to eligibility caused by immigration requirements. Further, several staff members reported that even for those who received food stamps, the assistance simply was insufficient to feed a family larger than three.

> N (staff): Just think about it, according to the guidelines, for a single person, they give 200 dollars a month. For *one* person. Do you think that's enough? To feed one person with 200 dollars, it's not. Especially these days, the food is increasing, so high, so badly.

Additionally, all clients surveyed were forced to use the NGO food pantry to supplement whatever foods they were able to purchase, whether or not they were eligible for formal food assistance. Unfortunately, the pantry is only able to offer the same amount of food per family, independently from the number of family members. This results on a great strain on the pantry, and on many local residents experiencing hunger.

> Researcher: When people come here, how much of their needs would you say it covers?
> N (staff): It depends on how big is the family, because everybody receives the same amount. The food we give away is for 1 or 2 days. If you have 6 members, it's one meal.
> Y (staff): We don't give a week's worth of groceries. None of us do. This is emergency food, to see you through the day. You know there is probably enough pasta or tuna, that you could stretch it out for a couple of days. But we are not the solution. Pantries were never, never meant to be the solution. [Still], if they didn't have the food pantry and food stamps, I don't know what they'd be eating.
> R (staff): I think they are going hungry. But they come here and they are very enthusiastic. A lot of them are really happy to have the food here.

Yet another important barrier to healthy eating was the type and conditions of work. Most client participants struggled with seasonal jobs related to agriculture or tourism and, regardless of the relative stability of different jobs, most held multiple jobs to make ends meet. At these jobs, breaks were extremely uncommon, even for meal times, which compounded the abuse of low-wages and unsafe conditions. As several participants noted:

> Y (staff): Our clients are abused. A lot. And taken advantage of. A lot. So, you know, they may not get paid even minimum wage, they may not get a lunch break, or any kind of break, you know. They are expected to work through. And some employers don't pay.
> R (staff): I hear from many clients that they have to get up at 2 or 3 in the morning. So [eating healthfully] is really difficult for them, because they won't have any markets close or by the time they get there, it's probably just the 7-11 that will be open. [Also] we just had a case where this guy had to get his finger amputated, because they didn't care for it from the cut.

Lastly, maybe the greatest barrier to healthy eating was the sheer constraints of poverty and competing basic needs. These competing needs often remained unmet, even in those cases in which clients were eligible for the range of means-tested social programs that they were able to sign up for with the assistance of NGO staff.

> Y (staff): You know, it's a full time job to be poor. For someone that, you know, immigration status isn't an issue, like say, lose their job, they have no savings, and they are living pay check to pay check. So then, they would come and say, let's apply for it all. And while we are waiting for your unemployment check to come, food stamps, and medical... let's sign you up, we have a contact too with PG&E, to sign people up for the care program, which is a discount.
> R (client): If your housing is good, you'll have a tighter budget for food. And if you choose a place with a lower rent, you will buy better food, but you will run the risk of living in a more dangerous neighborhood.
> L (client): And you will get sick because you'll be very uncomfortable, even if you eat well
> Researcher: So what happens when they find out that they can barely feed themselves?
> N (staff): They are trapped, you know. They have kids, they pay, they borrow.

Discussion

In our study, the barriers to healthy eating were structural rather than behavioral. By this, we do not wish to create a false dichotomy between structure (i.e., social relations, institutional arrangements, and social and economic policies) and human behavior. Rather, we mean that whatever knowledge about healthy eating and lifestyles participants did have, or however good their intentions to adopt those lifestyles appeared to be, structural constraints on behaviors, food-related or otherwise, made adopting healthy ones all but impossible.

Structural constraints to healthy eating included the high price of healthy foods (relative to income); the cost and inconvenience of transportation to well supplied and better-priced food outlets; language barriers between vendors in such outlets and study participants; the complexity of using food stamps at farmers' markets which recreated the stigma associated with the traditional paper format of food stamps; barriers to food assistance imposed by eligibility requirements related to immigration status; insufficient informal food assistance (e.g., food pantries) that could not guarantee either quantity or quality of foods; work conditions tied to precarious and low-paying employment that placed healthy eating out of participants' reach; and finally, competing basic needs and the sheer constraints of poverty, whereby participants were forced to choose among meeting their housing, nutritional, or other basic needs.

While our sample was small and non-random, and our study bears the interpretive limitations of qualitative research, it replicates a phenomenon illustrated in similar studies. For instance, Dinca-Panaitescu *et al.* (2011) have shown that low-income populations in Canada were more prone to suffering from diabetes, and when diagnosed, less able to prevent complications, despite having access to adequate diabetes care through the Canadian single-payer system. Participants reported difficulties following several of aspects of their diabetes treatment, including a healthy nutrition, because they could not afford them. The authors also found that the prevalence of diabetes in the lowest income group (less than $15,000 annual income) was 4.14 times higher than the highest income group (at least $80,000 annual income) – indeed, diabetes prevalence increased as income decreased – and that childhood poverty predicts adverse health outcomes, such as diabetes, in adulthood (Dinca-Panaitescu *et al.* 2011, Raphael 2011). Importantly, they also showed that the increasing awareness of the explosion of diabetes and of the SDH underpinning this explosion has not been accompanied by a concomitant effort by state actors and public health officials to act upon these factors, but rather by a redoubling of calls for lifestyle changes on a grand scale (Raphael *et al.* 2011).

The phenomenon of persistent blind spots in public discourses concerning diabetes and other health inequalities is consistent with the ideology of 'healthism', which, as Robert Crawford noted over 30 years ago, calls for individuals to take more responsibility for their health rather than rely on 'costly and inefficient' medical services. Then as now, this ideology is used to 'justify the retrenchment from rights and entitlements ... and to divert attention from the social causation of disease in the commercial and industrial sectors' (Crawford 1977, p. 663).

Healthism has roots in personal behavior theories of disease causation, which blossomed in the nineteenth century, and depoliticized disease by eschewing government's responsibility for the public's health and by turning it into an exclusively personal event. As Tesh (1988, p. 21) noted, much like current behavioral theories of disease, personal behavior theories 'not so much blamed the poor for their illness as ignored poverty altogether'. The assumption, Tesh (1988) noted, was that 'everyone already had the wherewithal to comply with the behavioral requirements for a healthy life' and that poor health was nothing but the result of 'inadequate health education and bad habits'. Thus, the author concluded, personal behavior theories of disease causation precluded any social and economic reforms in the pursuit of health and enshrined the values of laissez-fair capitalism – they were a 'homage to middle-class life' (Tesh 1988).

Our own research has shown that the ideology of personal responsibility is alive and well in the diabetes medical literature: even when this literature mentions factors such as poverty as barriers to diabetes prevention or care, or even includes them as predictors (i.e., potential causes), it largely relegates them to the background, or buries them in calls to redouble the efforts to encourage and empower poor communities to embrace healthy lifestyles within their restricted means (Chaufan 2006, Chaufan and Weitz 2009).

Nevertheless, as our study indicates, however effective health education and lifestyle interventions might be for particular individuals, they will not slow down the diabetes pandemic. Addressing the latter requires changes in public policies guaranteeing basic needs, including but not limited to healthy food choices. As Bell *et al.* (2011, P. 5) noted, from the perspective of health inequalities the rhetoric of 'individual choice' pervading contemporary public health conceals 'the unequal impact [of health inequalities] across the population'.

The combination of a re-emergence in communicable diseases and widespread under-nutrition on the one hand, and the dramatic rise in chronic non-communicable diseases such as diabetes on the other, has been called a 'paradox' (Zimmet 2003). Yet this combination is only a paradox if it is assumed that the former are due to poverty, while the latter are the result of 'abundance'. However, if it is recognized that disease rates and their unequal distribution are indicators of an unequal distribution of the SDH and of inequalities in social power generally, which remain the strongest predictors of ill-health even as their specific health manifestations change over time (Link and Phelan 1995), the paradox all but disappears.

In our view, public health professionals are ideally positioned and have the necessary legitimacy to advocate for policy changes that impinge on the SDH. However, for this to happen, a shift must occur among public health practitioners, who must recognize that there is no health-educational 'fix' to poverty, socioeconomic inequality, and political disenfranchisement. This shift could translate into research that tests theories and programs that acknowledge the role of the SDH in disease causation, practice that uses this knowledge to advocate for transforming structural conditions at their root, and a recognition of the limits of medical and public health institutions, accompanied by a professional and personal commitment to engage with other forms of praxis seeking to change the social and political contexts (Waitzkin and Britt 1989).

Acknowledgments

This study was funded by the School of Nursing at the University of California-San Francisco. We wish to thank the reviewers and editors for their useful feedback, and the staff and faculty at the Institute for Health and Aging, especially Professor Patrick Fox, without whose continuing support it would have been impossible to conduct this study.

References

Baker, D., 2007. Behind the gap between productivity and wage growth. *Center for Economic and Policy Research*, Issue Brief (February). Available from: http://www.cepr.net/documents/publications/0702_productivity.pdf [Accessed 25 March 2009].

Baker, D., 2010. Weak job growth pushes employment rate back to downturn low-point. *Center for Economic and Policy Research*, Issue Brief (December). Available from: http://www.cepr.net/index.php/data-bytes/jobs-bytes/2010-12 [Accessed 17 January 2011].

Barker, D.J.P., 2003. The developmental origins of adult disease. *European Journal of Epidemiology*, 18, 736–788.

Bell, K., Salmon, A., and McNaughton, D., 2011. Alcohol, tobacco, obesity and the new public health. *Critical Public Health*, 21 (1), 1–8.

Bernstein, J., McNichol, E., and Nicholas, A., 2000. Pulling apart: a state by state analysis of income trends. *Center on Budget and Policy Priorities, Economic Policy Institute*. Available from: http://www.cbpp.org/archiveSite/1-18-00sfp-part1.pdf [Accessed 17 January 2011].

Branca, F. and Ferrari, M., 2002. Impact of micronutrient deficiencies on growth: the stunting syndrome. *Annals of Nutrition and Metabolism*, 46 (Suppl. 1), 8–17.

Centers for Disease Control and Prevention (CDC), 2011. National diabetes fact sheet. Atlanta, Centers for Disease Control and Prevention. January 26. Available from: http://www.cdc.gov/diabetes/pubs/pdf/ndfs_2011.pdf [Accessed 1 February 2010].

Chaufan, C., 2006. *Sugar blues: issues and controversies concerning the type 2 diabetes epidemic.* Unpublished dissertation. Sociology, University of California, Santa Cruz. PhD Sociology (Philosophy), 367.

Chaufan, C., 2008. What does justice have to do with it? A bioethical and sociological perspective on the diabetes epidemic. *In*: B. Katz Rothman and E. Armstrong, eds. *Bioethical issues: sociological perspectives – advances in medical sociology*. New York: Elsevier, 269–300.

Chaufan, C., Davis, M., and Constantino, S., 2011. The twin epidemics of poverty and diabetes: understanding diabetes disparities in a low-income Latino and immigrant neighborhood. *Journal of Community Health*, DOI: 10.1007/s10900-011-9406-2.

Chaufan, C. and Weitz, R., 2009. The elephant in the room: the invisibility of poverty in research on type 2 diabetes. *Humanity and Society*, 33, 74–98.

Crawford, R., 1977. You are dangerous to your health: the ideology and politics of victim blaming. *International Journal of Health Services*, 7 (4), 663–680.

Commission on Social Determinants of Health (CSDH), 2008. Closing the gap in a generation: health equity through action on the social determinants of health – executive summary. Geneva, World Health Organization. Available from: http://whqlibdoc. who.int/hq/2008/WHO_IER_CSDH_08.1_eng.pdf [Accessed 13 February 2009].

Department of Health and Human Services (DHHS), 2003. *National agenda for public health action: the national public health initiative on diabetes and women's health.* Atlanta: Department of Health and Human Services, Centers for Disease Control and Prevention.

Diabetes Research Working Group, 1999. Conquering diabetes: a strategic plan for the 21st Century. Bethesda, NIH.

Dinca-Panaitescu, S., *et al.*, 2011. Diabetes prevalence and income: results of the Canadian Community Health Survey. *Health Policy*, 99 (2), 116–123.

Forssas, E., *et al.*, 2003. Widening socioeconomic mortality disparity among diabetic people in Finland. *European Journal of Public Health*, 13 (1), 38–43.

Irons, J.S., 2007. Typical families see income and earnings decline. *Economic Policy Institute.* Available from: http://www.epi.org/economic_snapshots/entry/webfeatures_ snapshots_20070905/ [Accessed 1 February 2011].

Jovanovic, L. and Pettitt, D.J., 2001. Gestational diabetes mellitus. *JAMA*, 286 (20), 2516–2518.

Link, B. and Phelan, J., 1995. Social conditions as fundamental causes of disease. *Journal of Health and Social Behavior*, 35, 80–94.

Mohanty, S.A., *et al.*, 2005. Health care expenditures of immigrants in the United States: a nationally representative analysis. *American Journal of Public Health*, 95 (8), 1431–1438.

Morikawa, Y., *et al.*, 1997. Ten-year follow-up study on the relation between the development of non-insulin-dependent diabetes mellitus and occupation. *American Journal of Industrial Medicine*, 31 (1), 80–84.

Naser, K.A., Gruber, A., and Thomson, G., 2006. The emerging pandemic of obesity and diabetes: are we doing enough to prevent a disaster? *International Journal of Clinical Practice*, 60 (9), 1093–1097.

Physicians for Human Rights, 2000. Hungry at home: a study of food insecurity and hunger among legal immigrants in the United States. ISBN 1-879707-30-6. Available from: http:// physiciansforhumanrights.org/library/report-hungerathome-2000.html [Accessed 17 January 2010].

Raphael, D., 2011. Poverty in childhood and adverse health outcomes in adulthood. *Maturitas*, 69 (1), 22–26.

Raphael, D., *et al.*, 2011. A toxic combination of poor social policies and programmes, unfair economic arrangements and bad politics: the experiences of poor Canadians with Type 2 diabetes. *Critical Public Health*, doi: 10.1080/09581596.2011.607797.

RealtyTrack – National Real Estate Trends. Available from: http://www.realtytrac.com/ trendcenter/ [Accessed 8 March 2011].

Seligman, H., *et al.*, 2007. Food insecurity is associated with diabetes mellitus: results from the National Health Examination and Nutrition Examination Survey (NHANES) 1999–2002. *Journal of General Internal Medicine*, 22 (7), 1018–1023.

Tesh, S.N., 1988. *Hidden arguments: political ideology and disease prevention policy.* New Brunswick and London: Rutgers University Press.

The Lancet,, 2011. The diabetes pandemic. *The Lancet*, 378 (9786), 99.

US Department of Agriculture, 2011. Supplemental Nutrition Assistance Program (SNAP) Annual Summary (January). Available from: http://www.fns.usda.gov/pd/ SNAPsummary.htm [Accessed 11 April 2011].

US Department of Commerce Economics and Statistics Administration US Census Bureau, 2010. Income, poverty, and health insurance coverage in the United States: 2009. Available from: http://www.census.gov/prod/2010pubs/p60-238.pdf [Accessed 23 September 2010].

US Department of Commerce Economics and Statistics Administration US Census Bureau, 2011. Income, poverty, and health insurance coverage in the United States: 2010. Available from: http://www.census.gov/prod/2011pubs/p60-239.pdf [Accessed 1 September 2011].

US Department of Housing and Urban Development, Affordable Housing. Available from: http://www.hud.gov/offices/cpd/affordablehousing/index.cfm [Accessed 1 February 2011].

UnitedHealth Center for Health Reform & Modernization, 2010. The United States of diabetes: Challenges and opportunities in the decade ahead, Working Paper 5. Minnetonka, MN: UnitedHealth Center for Health Reform & Modernization.

Waitzkin, H. and Britt, T., 1989. A critical theory of medical discourse: how patients and health professionals deal with social problems. *International Journal of Health Services*, 19 (4), 577–597.

White, R., Beech, B.M., and Miller, S., 2009. Health care disparities and diabetes care: practical considerations for primary care providers. *Clinical Diabetes*, 27 (3), 105–112.

Wright, G., 2003. Rising diabetes rates in Appalachia shock health officials. *Times Recorder*, Sunday, September 14. Available from: www.zanesvilletimesrecorder.com/news/stories/200330914/localnews/258613.html [Accessed 21 June 2004].

Zimmet, P., 2003. The burden of type 2 diabetes: are we doing enough? *Diabetes Metabolism*, 29, 6S19–6S18.

Blaming the consumer – once again: the social and material contexts of everyday food waste practices in some English households

David Evans

Sociology and the Sustainable Consumption Institute, University of Manchester, Oxford Road, M13 9PL, UK

In public debates about the volume of food that is currently wasted by UK households, there exists a tendency to blame the consumer or individualise responsibilities for affecting change. Drawing on ethnographic examples, this article explores the dynamics of domestic food practices and considers their consequences in terms of waste. Discussions are structured around the following themes: (1) feeding the family; (2) eating 'properly'; (3) the materiality of 'proper' food and its intersections with the socio-temporal demands of everyday life and (4) anxieties surrounding food safety and storage. Particular attention is paid to the role of public health interventions in shaping the contexts through which food is at risk of wastage. Taken together, I argue that household food waste cannot be conceptualised as a problem of individual consumer behaviour and suggest that policies and interventions might usefully be targeted at the social and material conditions in which food is provisioned.

Introduction

In the 2003 *Critical Public Health* special issue on food, Holm (2003) suggested that the concept of victim blaming – in which responsibility for (bad) individual health is assigned to the (wrong) decisions that individuals make – has relevance beyond critical discussions of public health policies. By way of example she suggests that debates about political consumerism – in which individuals are expected to solve social problems by altering the ways in which they consume – exhibit a parallel tendency to blame the consumer. Debates around the amount of food that is currently wasted by consumers in the UK are a case in point. It is estimated that UK households throw away roughly 1/3 of the food that they purchase for consumption (WRAP 2009) and public debates about food waste certainly appear to blame consumers[1] for their (assumed) profligacy and (imagined) lack of culinary competence.

By way of corrective, the analysis here offers a broadly sociological analysis of household food waste. I take a cue from work that critiques the individualisation of responsibilities – in public debates and policy interventions – for affecting changes in behaviour and/or consumption. There are identifiable threads of sociological engagement with issues of health promotion (Bunton *et al.* 1995) which provide a welcome rejoinder to approaches (see, e.g. Bettinghaus 1986) that seek to influence health-related behaviours through appeals to knowledge and attitudes. In addition to Foucauldian critiques of bodily discipline and the governmental imperatives of self-regulation (Peterson *et al.* 2010), existing researches have highlighted how 'knowledge-attitude-behaviour' interventions fail to recognise the complexity and dynamics of everyday life. For example, Ioannou's (2005) analysis of smoking, eating, drinking alcohol and exercise suggests that these activities should not be viewed as health-related behaviours but understood in relation to everyday issues. In this spirit, Lindsay (2010) demonstrates the role of food consumption in performing social identities and social relations and argues that informational campaigns do not adequately acknowledge the complex and contradictory concerns that individuals juggle as they make 'food choices' in their everyday lives. In terms of theorising these moves, Delormier *et al.* (2009) suggest that public health interventions in food consumption should conceive of eating not in terms of behaviour but as a social practice. Drawing on Giddens' (1984) structuration theory, they call for greater attention to social structure (rules and resources) in order to better understand the ways in which eating is embedded in the flow of day-to-day life (Delormier *et al.* 2009, p. 217).

Similar issues are being raised in debates around the environmental impacts of consumption and attendant policy approaches to 'behaviour change'. In a recent article, Shove (2010) criticises existing climate change policies for their reliance on individualist perspectives drawn from behavioural economics and social psychology. She suggests that these approaches are grounded in the ABC framework where:

> '"A" stands for attitude, "B" for behaviour and "C" for choice' (Shove 2010, p. 1274).

Against this, a distinctly sociological approach towards sustainable consumption and behaviour change has emerged that is grounded in various strands of practice theory (see Røpke 2009 for a useful overview). The idea here, briefly, is that at any point in time there exists an established set of understandings, procedures and engagements that govern appropriate conduct within a particular practice. In this perspective, consumption is not a practice *per se*; rather it occurs within, and for the sake of, practices and being a competent practitioner (Warde 2005, p. 137). Accordingly, consumption is theorised in relation to the dynamics of everyday life and the social organisation of practices (see, e.g. Shove 2003, Southerton *et al.* 2004, Watson 2008). It follows that initiatives and policies for sustainable consumption should not target individuals and choices; rather, they should focus on the social and material contexts through which practices are ordered and (re)produced (Southerton *et al.* 2009). These insights are taken here as a useful framework through which to discuss household food waste.

The debate about food waste in the UK

It is estimated (WRAP 2009) that UK households throw away 8.7 million tonnes of uneaten food each year and that at least 5.3 million tonnes are avoidable. The annual financial cost of this avoidable waste is estimated at £12 billion (£480 per household) and the environmental impact is equivalent to 20 million tonnes of carbon dioxide emissions.[2] Whilst prominent commentators (e.g. Stuart 2009) do not lay the blame solely at the door of consumers; public and policy imaginations are focused disproportionately on domestic waste. Within these debates, recommendations appear to be limited to interventions that target knowledge, attitudes and the behaviours that individuals choose to undertake. For example, Stuart (2009, p. 77) stresses the need to raise awareness of the 'non-financial costs of wasting food' (environmental impacts, world hunger). Similarly, WRAP's lovefoodhatewaste campaign[3] aims to raise awareness about the consequences of food waste and provide information that will help individuals to change their behaviour. These suggestions are refreshingly well-intentioned and non-judgemental; however, they continue to individualise responsibilities for affecting change and so miss the ways in which so-called 'waste behaviours' relate to the dynamics of everyday life. It is this tendency that initiated the study discussed below.

Before turning to the study, a brief note on terminology is required. I view waste as a consequence of how something is disposed as opposed to an innate characteristic of certain objects. In this view, surplus matter is not necessarily the same as waste insofar as it could conceivably be placed in conduits of disposal (Gregson *et al.* 2007) that save it from wastage. It follows that something is wasted when it is disposed of through a trajectory that connects it to the waste stream. The empirical work that informs this analysis found that surplus food was routinely disposed of through the waste stream via the bin (Evans forthcoming) as opposed to being handed down, handed around or otherwise saved from wastage (e.g. through composting).[4] For the purposes of the discussions that follow, then, surplus food is treated as synonymous with food waste. When referring to food, I refer only to that which could have been eaten – I am not referring to things that UK households tend not to eat (such as tea bags or apple cores) nor am I referring to things that are discarded in the preparation of food (such as fruit and vegetable peelings). Finally, for reasons of brevity and consistency – when referring to specific meals, I refer only to evening meals.

The study

The analysis that follows is based on a broadly ethnographic study in which I adopted a material culture approach to the research design (Evans 2011). The fieldwork involved 8 months (November 2009 to July 2010) of sustained and intimate contact with the residents and households encountered on two 'ordinary' streets – pseudonymously called Rosewall Crescent and Leopold Lane – in and around South Manchester. I use the term 'ordinary' to signal that the streets were chosen because, following Miller (2008), I had no particular reason to chose them other than attempting to encounter everyday lives as they are found without recourse to the categories of social/sociological analysis. As a study of material culture, the emphasis was on the logic of stuff itself (the passage of 'food' into 'waste') and not the reasons why particular 'types' of household waste food. Participants were recruited by dropping information leaflets through doors and following this up with successive rounds of door knocking. In total, 19 households participated in the study and whilst this sample is by no means representative, the heterogeneous nature of the areas in which I was working ensured a reasonable spread of income band, age, housing structure, housing tenure and household composition.

The study was undertaken to explore household food waste; however, I anticipated that a narrow focus on disposal would be problematic in terms of recruiting and retaining respondents. Moreover, in order to explore the passage of 'food' into 'waste', I decided to focus on the broader processes, dynamics and relations that accompany this movement. Accordingly, the study explored the ways in which households plan for and shop for food; how they prepare, consume and eat it; how they store it; and ultimately the ways in which they dispose of the food that they do not eat. In terms of carrying out the fieldwork, I utilised a range of qualitative of approaches. I conducted repeat in-depth interviews (Mason 2002) with respondents in which we discussed the various ways in which they shop for, prepare, eat, store and dispose of food. I also spent a lot of time 'hanging out' in respondents' homes, their streets and the areas in which the study took place. Additionally, I adopted a range of less familiar techniques. These included diary records; 'going along' (Kusenbach 2003) with participants as they shop for and prepare food; cupboard rummages and fridge inventories; and kitchen and home tours (Pink 2004).

Feeding the family

Throughout the study, respondents were found to routinely overprovision food such that they were often left with a certain amount of food that they struggled to then find a use for. Typically, this situation arose when a particular item of food was purchased for a specified purpose but the volume in which it could be purchased exceeded the volume required. For example, Julia is in her early 30s and lives with her husband and two young children on Rosewall Crescent. Talking though the items in her fridge, she explained:

> J: I got that to do a, a cauliflower cheese last week but I didn't need the whole thing um floret [...] and if I am honest, I don't really know what I'll do with it or can
>
> I: I see
>
> J: and [laughing] cauli just isn't the same without cheese, none of us really like it on its own without erm, yeah so there isn't anything we do that uses it [...] and I worry a lot, not being able to use the food that we have bought.

Such items are at risk of not being eaten and interventions targeted at reducing household food waste are sensitive to this predicament. For example, the lovefoodhatewaste campaign website has a 'recipes' section that gives suggestions on how to find a use for leftover ingredients.[5] For the respondents encountered in this study, however, the problem was not one of lacking knowledge about what to do with the food that needs using up. To the contrary, they had very clear ideas about how leftover ingredients might be saved from wastage, but were unable to put these ideas into practice given the domestic context in which they provision food. For example, Suzanne is a single mother in her 30s who lives on Rosewall Crescent with her two children. Going through her fridge, she discussed a bag of spinach with about ¼ of the contents remaining:

> S: If it was just me, it would be easy enough I would I dunno do something with it like omelette. Something quick that uses it up.
>
> I: If it was just you?

S: Yeah, I mean it would be it doesn't need to be great and I don't have to bother but my lot probably aren't going to be all that impressed if I put I spinach omelette down for their tea [laughs]

I: Why's that then?

S: for a start [laughing] they are fussy buggers [...] well I suppose that they do eat different things but it takes a while to get there as there is a definite, definitely prefer tried and tested recipes that they've had before and know they like.

In common with many respondents, Suzanne's food practices are located in a household context where the culinary repertoire is relatively fixed and provisioning highly routinised (DeVault 1991). It is well-understood that in feeding the family, the work of caring requires those responsible (usually women) to subsume their preferences to those of others within the household (DeVault 1991, Burridge and Barker 2009). Given that Suzanne's family are unlikely to be receptive to new introductions, especially 'improvised' foods that do not constitute a 'proper meal' (on which more below), it is perhaps not surprising that she would go for a 'tried and tested recipe' over something that would use the spinach up. However, as a consequence, this spinach was rendered obsolete and in turn, wasted.

Eating 'properly'

Just as the process of feeding the family is well-understood in terms of practising care and devotion towards significant others, it can also be noted that the provisioning of 'proper meals' has been identified as the appropriate means of doing so (Murcott 1983, Charles and Kerr 1988, Jackson 2009). The empirical material gathered here supports this idea. For example, Sarah lives on Rosewall Crescent and is a married mother of two in her early 30s. Having returned to work as a result of her youngest child starting school, she explained:

S: [b]efore I went back they always had good, proper food and ate well but it becomes a little bit harder to do when I am not at home so much and so what I do is spend Sunday cooking meals for the week ahead [...] and that doesn't stretch the whole week and but a night of junk food is alright and for the rest I try to mix proper things in with easy things.

The imperative to eat 'properly' also emerged in the accounts and experiences of those not living as part of a family (however defined), but in these cases, the emphasis was on healthy living (Peterson *et al.* 2010) and practising an ethic of caring for the self. For example, Pete is in his early 20s and living with 'a bunch of randoms' in a houseshare on Leopold Lane. Talking about how his work takes him 'on the road' a lot, he explained:

P: [i]t would be all to easy when you all over the shop to just pick up a takeaway or, god, there have been times that I've just survived on microwaved stuff from the garage but it's no good. You have to look after yourself, don't you and I don't want to turn into a fat bas- so yeah I now try and eat a bit better.

This of course raises the question of what constitutes 'proper' food and existing researches suggest that it is understood to encompass fresh, healthy ingredients that are used to prepare cooked meals from scratch whilst incorporating a variety of flavours and ethnic cuisines (Douglas 1972, Murcott 1983, Charles and Kerr 1988, Mitchell 1999, Bugge and Almas 2006, Short 2006, Halkier 2009). Again, the empirical material gathered here suggests that respondents recognised these as appropriate procedures and engagements with practices of food provisioning. The following excerpt from my field diary is drawn from a Sunday that I spent with Sarah as she prepared meals for the upcoming week:

> *Sarah opens up the fridge and announces that it looks right and good to have all of these fresh ingredients in and she sets about moving some ingredients [peppers, lean steak mince, garlic] over to the chopping board. These are joined by onions and a carrot from the cupboard. She tells me how she is going to cook a lasagne as that can easily be put in the fridge and reheated 'on the night' and served with a salad to create a proper meal in minutes [...] she chops up all three peppers in the packet and I ask if she is planning to use them all in the lasagne to which she replies that she is chopping them ready to be used in a Moroccan dish that she is going to cook later and here she explains that it is important that they have something 'lighter' and 'healthier' in the week and that her children should have exposure to flavours from other cultures.* (Field diary March 2010)

These understandings and definitions of 'proper food' were also recognised by respondents who did not themselves adhere to the attendant procedures and engagements. For example, Ceri is a single mother of three and is in her early 20s. She lives on Rosewall Crescent in a housing trust home. The following extract from my field diary is drawn from an occasion when I accompanied her to the supermarket:

> *As we walk down the frozen food aisle, she tells me that this is where she fills her trolley up. She jokes about how she doesn't really pick up much in the fruit and veg aisle. Various freezer doors are opened and frozen chips, fish fingers, pizzas and pies go into her trolley. She looks at me and tells me that she knows that I think it is all ok but also states that she feels like a 'first rate failure'. I ask her why and she says that she feels like one of those people 'doing it all wrong on the Jamie Oliver show'. With this she tells me that she knows that she should be cooking like he suggests but points out that it isn't 'how her life is' and she can't 'live up to it' [...] Moving down the aisle a little, she picks up lots of frozen vegetables and jokes that even when she cooks right, she cheats.* (Field diary June 2010)

Not only does Ceri define her own food practices in relation to dominant understandings of competence, but she also appears very troubled by not 'living up' to them.

It is instructive to note that biomedical interventions in health promotion – such as healthy living guidelines (Lindsay 2010) – play a role in shaping these definitions of proper food. For example, fresh fruits and vegetables were positioned as good, whilst processed foods that are high in salt or sugar were seen as bad. Without wishing to comment on the legitimacy or nutritional significance of these expectations, they can be viewed as helping to shape the routines in which households end up wasting food. Notably, a lot of 'proper' food is perishable and so at risk of being wasted if it is not eaten within a particular timeframe. Viewed as such, the materiality of foodstuffs themselves assume importance in terms of organising the practices through which they must be used or otherwise wasted.

Materiality and temporality

This section considers waste as a consequence of the ways in which the materiality of food intersects with the broader socio-temporal context of food practices. Where public debates intimate that food waste arises when individuals do not have enough time to cook 'properly', the respondents encountered here reveal a more subtle mismatch between the materiality of food and the rhythms of everyday life.

For example, Tamsin is in her mid-20s and lives alone on Leopold Lane. She explained that she tries to eat properly but that this often involves buying '5 different ingredients' for a particular recipe and that these are not available in quantities that are suitable for a single person living on her own. Additionally, she explained how her employment requires her to travel away from Manchester frequently such that she 'does not know where she is going to be from one moment to the next':

> T: So when I go away, right, I simply have no memory um recollection of what's going on in my fridge [. . .] so when I get back into Manchester, the train gets in and all I really know is that I am tired and hungry and in desperate need of food
>
> I: so what do you do?
>
> T: Well, generally one of two things. Either I go for something quick and easy from the local supermarket – perhaps a ready meal and a bagged up salad or if it's the weekend, I can justify a cheeky takeaway [. . .]
>
> I: [. . .] and what about the ingredients that you already had in
>
> T: um, well very often I end up not getting to make anything from them before they are too far gone [. . .] it's actually very hard to stay on top of it all.

The problem of keeping on top of ingredients in various states of decay was not exclusive to persons living alone and managing an erratic work schedule. Respondents who provisioned food within a family context were found to do so at relatively fixed intervals, typically every 7–10 days. Even allowing for the proliferation of 'mini' supermarkets where 'bits and bobs' could be picked up 'as and when', the vast majority of grocery shopping tended to be acquired via a 'big shop' at a large out of town supermarket. Through going along with participants on these shopping trips, I discovered that they tended to buy roughly the same things at each visit. Whilst very few households planned what would be eaten meal by meal, there was certainly a tacit expectation that certain dishes would be eaten (recalling the preference for a relative fixed culinary repertoire) at some point within the period between visits (see also DeVault 1991). However, these habituated routines of food provisioning were easily thrown out of balance by the rather more fluid nature of the ways in which lives are lived. As Julia explained:

> J: There is always something gets in the way of what I was going to d-
>
> I: you plan out what you are going to eat each night?
>
> J: um- I suppose no, not but I think I have a sense of what I might do throughout the week
>
> I: sorry, I just threw you right off [laughing] – you were saying that something always gets in the way
>
> J: oh, um, yeah like if I know I've some greens that need using – I'll think I can do them with some chops or wh- you know one night in the week [. . .] but other things always come up
>
> I: like?
>
> J: oh god, anything like if there is something on at school or one of us has something else on we might not have what I was thinking.

She went on to explain what would happen to the 'greens' that ended up not being eaten:

> J: If they don't get used before a new bag comes in they will go
>
> I: thrown out?
>
> J: bad but they go when the new ones come in

I: why is that?

J: well they didn't get used and I am definitely not going to use them if there is a newer pack that I could, um, need to use before that starts getting old.

In this example, food gets displaced and wasted as a result of a mismatch between the food that is provisioned and the food that is eaten within a given period of 7–10 days. Again, the lovefoodhatewaste campaign is attuned to this situation and gives advice on planning meals such that they mirror more closely the food that is provisioned when going shopping.[6] However, this advice is not sensitive to the temporal dynamics of everyday life nor does it appear to recognise that the materiality of food (and the temporalities of its decay) render it unable to accommodate disruptions to household provisioning routines.

Of course, it might reasonably be assumed that the domestic freezer might operate as a 'time machine' (Shove and Southerton 2000) to help households circumvent some of the tensions created at the intersection of food's materiality and the rhythms of everyday life. However, food that is well-suited to the freezer tended to be viewed as undesirable on the grounds that it does not constitute 'proper' food. For example, in discussing the amount of work she does on Sundays to ensure that her family eat 'properly', Sarah pointed out that:

S: It would definitely be easier if I was one of those Mums that go to Iceland[7] [laughing] you know, getting all that stuff for a fiver . . . god, would save loads of money and I bet I wouldn't ever chuck anything out as that stuff is pumped so full of crap that it never goes off

I: you are never tempted to start doing that?

S: um maybe but I never would, couldn't um I wouldn't give that to my family as it isn't food

I: how would you feel about frozen vegetables then?

S: they are better but really they can't compare to fresh.

In this example – and throughout the study – the refusal of certain foodstuffs extends beyond concerns about eating healthily to incorporate class-based processes of classification and distinction on the grounds of taste in food (Warde 1997). More generally, it is instructive to highlight that the imperative to eat 'properly' (discussed above) leads to the provisioning of foodstuffs that are at risk – against the backdrop of the routines and rhythms discussed in this section – of wastage. Viewed as such, a picture of household food waste as the fall out of everyday life begins to emerge.

Food risk and anxiety

This section picks up on the idea that food waste arises as a consequence of households juggling the complex and contradictory demands of day-to-day living. In addition to the aforementioned concerns about healthy and 'proper' eating; the respondents encountered were found to be negotiating concerns about food safety and storage. Throughout the study, respondents were quite explicit that once food has 'past its best', it is no longer fit for human consumption and as such, should be cast as 'waste'.[8] There is not the space here to discuss the ways in which respondents evaluated food as 'past its best' but suffice to say, the processes and practices varied across households and according to foodstuff. For example, some households observed dates and labels stringently, whilst others rejected them in favour of 'trusting their nose'. Some evaluated food according to its aesthetic qualities ('it's gone all wrinkly') whilst others used *ad hoc* knowledge about how long it had been 'kicking about'. Some foodstuffs were positioned as highly risky (meat, poultry, fish and dairy) whilst others were thought to be more 'forgiving' with their riskiness limited to the potential for a decline in quality (onions, herbs and spices). Others still were thought to be salvageable in the sense that signs of being past their best could be removed to prevent the rest of the item being contaminated (e.g. cutting mould out off a corner to rescue a block of cheese). The unifying feature across households and in respect of all foodstuffs was an acute awareness that food harbours the potential to make people ill and that this risk accelerated evaluations of food as past its best. For example, Faye is in her late 20s and living with her boyfriend on Leopold Lane. Narrated retrospectively, she discussed some chicken breasts that they had thrown out the previous week:

> F: It costs doesn't it and well something died for that and we didn't eat it [...] such a waste. Not good.
>
> I: how come it didn't get eaten?
>
> F: just kind of forgot about it and to be honest yeah, when I came to it I thought it had been there are while so I thought to check the date
>
> I: was it in date?
>
> F: No it was probably a few something like a few days gone so I ummed and ahhed about it but it's chicken so you've got to be careful
>
> I: uh huh
>
> F: and I wasn't going to risk it as you're going to know about it if you eat bad chicken.

Similarly, Natalie is a divorcee in her mid-40s who lives on Rosewall Crescent with her two teenage children. Whilst talking about the items in her kitchen, I asked her about a saucepan that was on the stove:

> N: That's from stew that I made a few nights ago [...] I meant to put it in the fridge after it cooled, you know, and then have it another night [...] but it's probably not safe to eat as its been out for a few days now [...] crap, I really hate wasting food.

Both Faye and Natalie – in contrast to claims that modern consumers are anomalously profligate – are troubled by their acts of wasting food. More generally, virtually, every respondent informed me that 'it is wrong to waste food' and that they 'felt awful' about the instances in which they end up doing so. However, this section has shown that, again, biomedical interventions in health promotion are also being played out in the everyday lives of the households encountered here. It is instructive to note that throughout this study, discourses of food safety tended to 'win out' over anxieties about wasting food such that the imperative to ensure that unsafe food is not eaten appeared to provide adequate justification for acts of binning and wasting. It is certainly not my intention to question the legitimacy of concerns about food safety and storage, I am simply illustrating how they help create the context in which food is evaluated as past its best and consequently, constituted as waste.

Discussion

The preceding analysis does not dispute that current volumes of household food waste are problematic in a number of registers (developmental, environmental, financial). It does, however, suggest that it is overly simplistic to blame consumers for these problems or individualise responsibilities for solving them. Returning to the

ABC framework it would be wrong, on the evidence here, to suggest that there is a need for attitudinal change insofar as the respondents encountered did not appear to have a careless or callous disregard for the food that they end up wasting. More generally, the analysis has demonstrated some of the ways in which waste is a consequence of the ways in which domestic food practices are socially organised. I have focused specifically on the role of biomedical interventions in health promotion (food safety and storage, healthy eating) but more generally, I have paid attention to the broader social (family relations, socio-temporal context, tastes) and material (domestic technologies, the organic vitality of food, infrastructures of provision) conditions through which food is provisioned. Taken together, it seems somewhat perverse to position food waste as a matter of individuals making negative choices to engage in behaviours that lead to the wastage of food. Indeed, the analysis here suggests that food waste arises as a consequence of households negotiating the contingencies of everyday life and as such, it recalls those who critique biomedical models of health promotion (Ioannou 2005, Lindsay 2010).

It has not been my intention to systematically evaluate existing policies or interventions and the prescription of alternatives based on the small-scale exploratory analysis offered here is necessarily beyond the scope of this article. However, if pushed, I would be inclined to suggest that interventions in the material context of food practices are key. For example, if food was to be made readily available in different quantities (material infrastructures of provision), then the respondents encountered here may well end wasting less. Similarly, there may be some mileage in targeting the material properties of food itself by, for example, finding ways to normalise the provisioning of foodstuffs that are not susceptible to rapid decay. These recommendations are of course mere speculation and the take home message here is that any effort to reduce household food waste could usefully reach beyond the default position of blaming the consumer in order to target the social and material contexts through which food practices might be changed.

Acknowledgements

This research was made possible through funding from the Sustainable Consumption Institute at the University of Manchester. Additional writing was undertaken whilst I was a visiting researcher on the Economic and Social Research Council funded 'Waste of the World' programme (RES000232007). I thank Ulla Gustafsson, Liza Draper and Wendy Wills for their helpful guidance and editorial steer. I also thank the two anonymous referees whose useful and insightful comments have no doubt strengthened this article. The usual disclaimers apply. Above all, I am indebted to those who accommodated my sustained presence in their homes during the course of the fieldwork.

Notes

1. This is not victim blaming insofar as the 'victims' are not UK households but those in less developed countries (Stuart 2009).
2. The same impact as the emissions generated by ¼ of the cars on UK roads.
3. http://www.lovefoodhatewaste.com [Accessed 8 June 2011].
4. I am not claiming that households never do these things; I am simply highlighting the normativity of binning surplus food.
5. http://www.lovefoodhatewaste.com/recipes [Accessed 3 February 2011].
6. http://www.lovefoodhatewaste.com/save_time_and_money/two_week_menu [Accessed 7 February 2011].

7. Iceland is a food retailer in the UK that specialises in low-cost frozen foods.
8. Or more accurately, it is cast as excess at which point it is deemed appropriate to dispose of it through the waste stream (Evans forthcoming).

References

Bettinghaus, E., 1986. Health promotion and the knowledge-attitude-behaviour continuum. *Preventive Medicine*, 15, 475–491.

Bugge, A. and Almas, R., 2006. Domestic dinner: representations and practices of a proper meal among young suburban mothers. *Journal of Consumer Culture*, 6 (2), 203–228.

Bunton, R., Nettleton, S., and Burrows, R., eds., 1995. *The sociology of health promotion: critical analyses of consumption, lifestyle and risk*. London: Routledge.

Burridge, J. and Barker, M., 2009. Food as a medium for emotional management of the family: avoiding complaint and producing love. *In*: P. Jackson, ed. *Changing families, changing food*. Basingstoke: Palgrave Macmillan, 146–164.

Charles, N. and Kerr, M., 1988. *Women, food and families*. Manchester: Manchester University Press.

Delormier, T., Frohlich, K., and Potvin, L., 2009. Food and eating as social practice – understanding eating patterns as social phenomena and implications for public health. *Sociology of Health and Illness*, 31 (2), 215–228.

DeVault, M., 1991. *Feeding the family: the social organization of caring as gendered work*. Chicago, IL: Chicago University Press.

Douglas, M., 1972. *Implicit meanings*. London: Routledge.

Evans, D., 2011. Beyond the throwaway society: ordinary domestic practice and a sociological approach to household food waste. *Sociology* (awaiting issue). DOI: 10.1177/0038038511416150.

Evans, D., forthcoming. Binning, gifting and recovery: the conduits of disposal in household food consumption. *Environment and Planning D: Society and Space*.

Giddens, A., 1984. *The constitution of society*. Cambridge: Polity Press.

Gregson, N., Metcalfe, A., and Crewe, L., 2007. Moving things along: the conduits and practices of divestment in consumption. *Transactions of the Institute of British Geographers*, 32 (2), 187–200.

Halkier, B., 2009. Suitable cooking? Performance and positionings in cooking practices among Danish women. *Food, Culture and Society*, 12 (3), 357–377.

Holm, L., 2003. Blaming the consumer: on the free choice of consumers and the decline in food quality in Denmark. *Critical Public Health*, 13 (2), 139–154.

Ioannou, S., 2005. Health logic and health-related behaviours. *Critical Public Health*, 15 (3), 263–273.

Jackson, P., ed., 2009. *Changing families, changing food*. Basingstoke: Palgrave Macmillan.

Kusenbach, M., 2003. Street phenomenology: the go-along as ethnographic research tool. *Ethnography*, 4 (3), 455–485.

Lindsay, J., 2010. Healthy living guidelines and the disconnect with everyday life. *Critical Public Health*, 20 (4), 475–487.

Mason, J., 2002. Qualitative interviewing: asking, listening and interpreting. *In*: T. May, ed. *Qualitative research in action*. London: Sage, 225–241.

Miller, D., 2008. *The comfort of things*. Cambridge: Polity Press.

Mitchell, J., 1999. The British main meal in the 1990s: has it changed its identity?. *British Food Journal*, 101 (11), 871–883.

Murcott, A., 1983. It's a pleasure to cook for him: food, mealtimes and gender in some South Wales households. *In*: E. Garmarnikow, ed. *The public and the private*. London: Heinemann.

Peterson, A., *et al.*, 2010. Healthy living and citizenship: an overview. *Critical Public Health*, 20 (4), 391–400.

Pink, S., 2004. *Home truths: gender, domestic objects and everyday life*. Oxford: Berg.

Røpke, I., 2009. Theories of practice – new inspiration for ecological economic studies on consumption. *Ecological Economics*, 68, 2490–2497.

Short, F., 2006. *Kitchen secrets: the meaning of cooking in everyday life*. Oxford: Berg.

Shove, E., 2003. *Comfort, cleanliness and convenience – the social organisation of normality*. Oxford: Berg.

Shove, E., 2010. Beyond the ABC: climate change policy and theories of social change. *Environment and Planning A*, 42 (6), 1273–1285.

Shove, E. and Southerton, D., 2000. Defrosting the freezer: from novelty to convenience. A narrative of normalization. *Journal of Material Culture*, 5 (3), 301–319.

Southerton, D., Chappells, H., and Van Vliet, B., eds., 2004. *Sustainable consumption: the implications of changing infrastructures of provision*. London: Edward Elgar.

Southerton, D., McMeekin, A., and Evans, D., 2009. *International review of behaviour change initiatives*. Available from: http://www.scotland.gov.uk/Publications/2011/02/01104638/0 [Accessed 7 February 2011].

Stuart, T., 2009. *Waste: uncovering the global food scandal*. London: Penguin.

Warde, A., 1997. *Consumption, food and taste*. Cambridge: Polity.

Warde, A., 2005. Consumption and theories of practice. *Journal of Consumer Culture*, 5 (2), 131–153.

Watson, M., 2008. The materials of consumption. *Journal of Consumer Culture*, 8 (1), 5–10.

WRAP, 2009. *Household food and drink waste in the UK*. Available from: http://www.wrap.org.uk/retail/case_studies_research/report_household.html [Accessed 7 February 2011].

Health improvement, nutrition-related behaviour and the role of school meals: the usefulness of a socio-ecological perspective to inform policy design, implementation and evaluation

Sue N. Moore, Simon Murphy and Laurence Moore

Cardiff School of Social Sciences, Cardiff Institute of Society and Health, Cardiff University, 1-3 Museum Place, Cardiff CF10 3BD, UK

Schools have the potential to support children's learning of nutrition-related behaviours through their experiences with school food. The transformation of school meal programmes have featured within policies in the UK and the USA. However, such policies are at risk of not meeting their objectives as many children remain unwilling to consume healthier food. Socio-ecological health improvement frameworks emphasise the importance of assessing health needs and designing/evaluating policies by considering processes operating at policy, community, organisational and inter/intra-personal levels. This article explores the usefulness of the socio-ecological perspective as: a theoretical framework to assess health policy and needs; a methodological framework to inform the design of associated research; and an evaluative framework for policy implementations. This is achieved by demonstrating how a socio-ecological perspective was deployed during an exploratory study into the role of primary school dining halls in improving children's nutrition-related behaviour. This study revealed how policies at local and school levels reflected national objectives with respect to nutritional guidelines, but were also influenced by multiple, competing interests at other socio-ecological levels. These included pupils' food preferences; organisational objectives such as protecting school meal uptake; and the practices of school meal staff. It is argued that higher level policy interventions may have limited effectiveness if undermined by lack of attention to lower level factors. The use of socio-ecological frameworks as theoretical, methodological and evaluative tools to support a consistent, holistic approach during the design, implementation and evaluation of health improvement policies is recommended.

Background

Over the past two decades, deteriorating nutrition-related behaviour and increasingly sedentary lifestyles together with their association with increased morbidity and mortality have attracted attention on a global scale (World Health Organisation 2003). In particular, nutrition-related behaviour has been associated with cancer (World Cancer Research Fund 2007), cardiovascular disease (National Institute for Health and Clinical Excellence 2010), and the prevalence of obesity (Chaudhury *et al.* 2008) which is itself a risk factor for cardiovascular disease (McGee and Diverse populations collaboration 2005), stroke and type 2 diabetes (World Health Organisation 2003). Behavioural risk factors associated with health have an impact throughout the lives of individuals, and a more profound impact the earlier they are exhibited (World Health Organisation 2003). The associated challenges to public health have concerned policymakers both globally and nationally, including those within UK central government (Department of Health 2005) and the devolved governments of Scotland (Scottish Executive 2004) and Wales (Food Standards Agency Wales 2003).

In England and Wales, by the age of 11, children eat less fruit than nearly all their European counterparts (Currie *et al.* 2008). In the UK, during 2008–2009, children aged 4–18 years received 16–17% of their daily energy intake from sugar, which, although a downward trend, remains in excess of the dietary reference value (DRV) of 11% (Food Standards Agency and Department of Health 2010). During the same period, although total fat intake continued to approximate to the DRV of 35% per day, 12.9% of this was in the form of saturated fatty acids, for which the DRV is 11% per day. Childhood nutrition also exhibits social inequalities in that poor nutrition is strongly associated with social deprivation (Armstrong *et al.* 2003), as is the prevalence of childhood obesity.

By age 11 years, the levels of childhood obesity in the UK are 20% (Wales), 18% (Scotland) and 12% (England), compared to 14% worldwide (Currie *et al.* 2008). Only England and Scotland have sufficient data to illustrate trends in child weight. In Scotland, these data are suggestive of no further increases in excess weight (The Scottish Government 2010), and in England, childhood obesity appears to be stabilising (The Health and Social Care Information Centre 2010). However, amongst white children aged 5–10 years, disparities are evident in that obesity levels are not stabilising in the lower socio-economic groups (Stamatakis *et al.* 2010). Furthermore, childhood obesity is considered to be one of the greatest challenges to child health in the twenty-first century (Wardle 2005) as well as being a strong predictor of adult obesity (Deshmukh-Taskar *et al.* 2006).

Whilst there are several theories relating to the development of human behaviour over the lifespan (Dworetzky 1995), ecological theorists offer a holistic explanation (McLaren and Hawe 2005). Ecological Systems Theory (EST) espouses that human development is shaped by a number of systems or contexts (Bronfenbrenner 1979, 1986). These are: (1) the *micro-system* – the immediate settings in which an individual participates (e.g. home, school, workplace) and face-to-face inter-relations within them; (2) the *meso-system* – inter-relations between the settings in which the individual participates; (3) the *exo-system* – inter-relations between settings in which the person does not participate but which affect the immediate environment (e.g. the education system); (4) the *macro-system* – generalised patterns that define the substance and structure of other systems (e.g. societies, social groups) but which are modifiable (e.g. by public policy); and (5) the *chrono-system* – the passage of time, which recognises the cumulative effect of developmental transitions and dynamic relationships between contexts and individuals. This inter-relation between individuals and environments is central to the philosophy of social ecology (McLaren and

Hawe 2005). It is also evident within public health policies which emphasise the development of individuals' health-related skills within supportive environments (World Health Organisation 1986, 1991, 1997), one example of which is the health promoting school.

Socio-ecological health improvement frameworks

The concept of the health promoting school originated from the Ottawa Charter (World Health Organisation 1986), which identified schools as a potential public health setting (Parsons *et al.* 1996). Indeed, the potential of the health promoting school to influence nutrition-related behaviours in order to prevent mortality from diseases associated with eating unhealthily is regarded as critical (World Health Organisation 2009). The health promoting school operates at many of the levels espoused by EST by promoting the health of the staff, families, communities and pupils associated with it (World Health Organisation 2009). However, school-based health promotion initiatives have not always encompassed all the levels within EST in that they frequently incorporate processes within and between the most proximal levels (e.g. classroom, home or community) (Lister-Sharp *et al.* 1999) but exclude policy contexts (Mukoma and Flisher 2004). Similarly, policy has not always accounted for all influences within the EST model (Stronach *et al.* 2002) and policy evaluations have generally failed to recognise the multi-level complexity inherent within a health promoting school (Lister-Sharp *et al.* 1999, Mukoma and Flisher 2004). The socio-ecological health promotion framework proposed by McLeroy *et al.* (1988) is based upon EST and identifies multiple, inter-related leverage or evaluative points at policy, community, organisational, inter-personal and intra-personal levels that can be used to address such issues.

The aim of this article is to explore the usefulness of the socio-ecological perspective as conceptualised by McLeroy *et al.* (1988) as: (1) a theoretical framework to assess health policy and needs; (2) a methodological framework to inform the design of associated research studies; and (3) an evaluative framework for policy implementations. This is achieved by demonstrating how the socio-ecological perspective was applied within an exploratory study into the role of primary school dining halls in Wales in improving children's (age 4–11 years) nutrition-related behaviour.

Social ecology as a theoretical framework

From a theoretical perspective, socio-ecological analyses of literature relating to health needs, and health improvement policy approaches and their implementation can be used to construct models of the multi-level relationships and processes involved. Such models symbolise existing socio-ecological relationships and processes, and facilitate the identification of knowledge gaps where further research is suggested. In the case of the role played by school dining halls in influencing children's nutrition-related behaviour, the model shown in Figure 1 was constructed from a literature review and subsequently used to define a set of research questions.

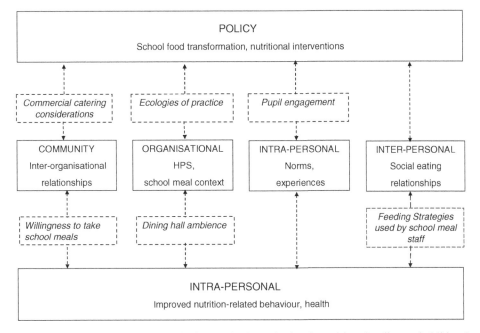

Figure 1. Theoretical socio-ecological organisation of school nutritional policy and children's nutrition-related behaviour. Dotted lines represent theoretical relationships between socio-ecological levels. Italicised text represents socio-ecological processes where further research is required.

Social ecology and health improvement policy

At the policy level, health improvement initiatives can be thought of as socio-ecological processes that seek to trigger other processes, such as behaviour modification, within the individual (i.e. at the intra-personal level). For example, education about healthy eating is a statutory requirement in Wales and Scotland (Welsh Government 2008b, Learning and Teaching Scotland 2009). However, education alone has been shown to be ineffective in influencing children's nutrition-related behaviour (Gould *et al.* 2006). On the other hand, the 'whole school' approach to education adopted within health promoting schools builds children's knowledge, skills, behaviours and attitudes through their experiences within the school context as well as the curriculum (Parsons *et al.* 1996). Indeed, consideration of the complementary role of the school meal service is an essential criterion for formal membership of the network of health promoting schools in the UK (Health Education Board for Scotland *et al.* 1996). Furthermore, the transformation of the school meal service, particularly with respect to the nutritional content of school meals, has been a prominent feature of policy agendas both within the UK (Scottish Executive 2002, School Meals Review Panel 2005, Welsh Government 2010) and the USA (US Department of Agriculture 2011). In the UK, reciprocal relationships are also evident between the policy and intra-personal levels in the form of pupil consultation mechanisms such as School Nutrition Action Groups (SNAGs) (Scottish Executive 2002, School Meals Review Panel 2005, Welsh Government 2008a). Nevertheless, indications are that even if nutritionally balanced meals are available, some children may not consume them (Gatenby 2007).

At the organisational level, further processes associated with the structures required for policy implementation mediate socio-ecological relationships between the policy and intra-personal levels (i.e. the influence of policy on behaviour and vice versa). For example, the provision of school meals in the UK falls within the remit of Local Education Authorities (LEAs) and is subject to compulsory, competitive tendering (Morgan 2006). This multi-layering of organisational involvement is a common feature of programmes that originate at national level (Coffield et al. 2007). It illustrates the complex web of inter-relationships between hierarchical layers of national and local government, and also between commercial providers. In addition, the original programme is potentially subjected to additional priorities at each decision making level. For example, competitive tendering is associated with a reduced focus on diet and health, and an increased focus on cost control and income generation (Davies 2005). Furthermore, the internal characteristics of the organisation are equally as important as its external relationships. For example, associations have been reported between the existence of school food policies and food availability (Rasmussen et al. 2006), which then influence the uptake of school meals and children's choices at the point of service (Paisley et al. 2006).

At the intra-personal level, nutritional interventions have typically sought to increase fruit and vegetable (F/V) consumption (Horne et al. 2004, Hendy et al. 2005, Bere et al. 2006, Day et al. 2008). From a health improvement perspective, it is clear from epidemiological data that F/V consumption can protect against chronic diseases such as cancer or heart disease. However, the strength of the relationship between the policy and intra-personal level has been undermined by the limited success of many previous nutritional interventions (Ciriza et al. 2008, de Sa and Lock 2008). This may be attributable to barriers operating at the intra-personal level in that the behaviour modification techniques used have generally been theoretically informed by Social Cognitive Theory (SCT) (Bere et al. 2006) despite the fact that its explanatory power for children is not understood (Resnicow et al. 1997). As cognitive maturation spans at least 12 years of the child's life (Dworetzky 1995), this suggests the importance of identifying behavioural modification processes that are both age-appropriate and theoretically informed.

In summary, a top-down socio-ecological analysis (i.e. from policy level to intra-personal level), suggests that processes at the policy, community, organisational and intra-personal levels may be inhibiting health improvement objectives. On the other hand, promising results have been obtained from an intervention in the USA where the social interactions between children and staff serving school meals have been used as opportunities to encourage children's fruit consumption (Schwartz 2007). The ability of current school-based nutritional policies to achieve their behavioural and health improvement objectives could arguably be improved were they to trigger such inter-personal processes. This suggests the importance of considering policy initiatives *in conjunction with* what has been learned about the processes involved in influencing nutrition-related behaviour, and how these are known to operate at other socio-ecological levels.

Social ecology and children's nutrition-related behaviour

From a socio-ecological perspective, although human behaviour is located at the intra-personal level, processes within and between all socio-ecological levels are important in fashioning this behaviour. For example, research has shown that children *learn* to eat during the transition from a diet of milk in infancy to an adult, omnivorous diet (Birch 1998) and that food preferences are relatively malleable until age 7 (Kelder *et al.* 1994). However, Piagetian theory would suggest that children may not be able to undertake the cognitive work required to associate food-related knowledge with potential eating outcomes (e.g. health) in order to make effective choices as their thoughts are based directly upon objects rather than hypotheses (Piaget and Inhelder 1969). Learning mechanisms that have been associated with eating are operant conditioning, classical conditioning and social learning which involve processes at the inter-personal level in the form of the feeding strategies used by caregivers during social eating interactions (Birch 1998). Strategies such as modelling (Hendy and Raudenbush 2000), repeated taste exposure (Birch and Marlin 1982), coercion (Fisher and Birch 1999, Fisher *et al.* 2002) and encouragement (Stark *et al.* 1986) have been shown to reliably influence nutrition-related behaviour. It is known that these strategies are used by parents in the home (Moore *et al.* 2007) and that, in schools, lunchtime supervisors use strategies used with their own children (Pike 2010). However, little is known about the practices of school meal staff (both lunchtime supervisors and school cooks) either with respect to their influence on nutrition-related behaviour, or their role in the delivery of school meal policies.

At the organisational level, meanwhile, nutrition-related behaviour is further influenced by the physical (Stroebele and De Castro 2004) and temporal (School Food Trust 2007) organisation of the eating environment, for example, accommodation and length of lunchtime. The emphasis on lunchtime management and the promotion of healthy eating often outweighs the emphasis on lunchtime as a social event (Pike 2008, Daniel and Gustafsson 2010). These negative aspects of dining hall ambience can undermine well-intentioned nutritional/health policies, not least of all by discouraging the uptake of free school meals (Pike and Colquhoun 2009). Furthermore, socio-ecological health improvement approaches recognise the influence of individuals and groups acting at various levels (Stokols 1992) such that those who may not be the ultimate target of a policy may be involved in its implementation. The multi-layered processes whereby individual experiences and beliefs influence local policies and/or practices are referred to as 'ecologies of practice' (Stronach *et al.* 2002). These involve a commitment to ideologies or adaptations of best practice which can lead to a preferred style of working, or judgements of how best to engage with particular individuals or contexts that may be at odds with policy. Thus, the social, physical and temporal characteristics of school dining halls also have implications for nutrition-related behaviour and policy implementation.

In summary, a bottom-up socio-ecological analysis of nutrition-related behaviour (i.e. from the intra-personal level to the policy level) reveals both issues and opportunities associated with processes operating within and between higher socio-ecological levels. This suggests a need to better understand how these processes could be harnessed within nutritional policy. The theoretical logic model in Figure 1 is derived by superimposing the discrete top-down and bottom-up socio-ecological analyses of policy approaches and health needs. In this way, theoretical relationships and processes are revealed (indicated by the dotted arrows and italicised text in Figure 1) where exploratory research may further inform health improvement initiatives. In this regard, social ecology can also be useful as a methodological tool.

Social ecology as a methodological framework

Socio-ecological frameworks can be used to inform the selection of a research methodology, the research methods and the recruitment strategy (i.e. categories of potential participants and the most appropriate method(s) to be used for each category). For example, testing a theoretical logic model such as that presented in Figure 1 suggests an exploratory qualitative methodology. However, Grzywacz and Fuqua (2000) note that the strength of socio-ecological approaches in acknowledging contextual complexity is also a limitation since the 'everything affects everything' approach is problematic. To understand the *relative* importance of the socio-ecological processes involved, it may be necessary to control some of the known sources of variation. Therefore, the study scope needs to be clearly defined. Accordingly, for the exploratory study into the role of primary school dining halls in improving children's nutrition-related behaviour, a case study methodology was adopted focussing on primary schools (children aged 4–11 years) in one LEA in Wales. Furthermore, the socio-ecological processes of interest were defined within two research aims which emerged from the top-down and bottom-up analyses of the literature, respectively. Aim 1 focussed on processes at the community, organisational and intra-personal levels and their relationship with nutritional policy. It sought to understand the school meal context and its implications for nutritional policy and primary schoolchildren's nutrition-related behaviour. Aim 2 focussed on processes at the inter-personal level and their relationships with nutritional policy and nutrition-related behaviour. It sought to understand the techniques used by school meal staff during social interactions within the primary school meal setting which directly or indirectly impact upon children's nutrition-related behaviour.

Social ecology can further be used to inform the methods used. For example, observational methods allow data about the physical *and* social world to be gathered directly (Foster 1996) allowing the dynamic relationships between context and individual that are central to the philosophy of social ecology (McLaren and Hawe 2005) to be captured. However, social actions are both performed *and* talked about, requiring the meanings they elicit to be super-imposed rather than juxtaposed (Atkinson *et al.* 2003). Therefore, consideration of the use of methods which complement observation, such as interviewing, is important. Consequently, the methods used within the exploratory study included dining hall observations, semi-structured interviews, and focus groups. Full details of this study have been previously reported (Moore *et al.* 2010, 2010a, 2010b).

Finally, social ecology can be used to inform the recruitment strategy in order to identify potential participants at each socio-ecological level, and then the most appropriate research method(s) for each type of participant. Figure 2 illustrates how this was achieved. Potential participants were identified at each socio-ecological level as appropriate for each research aim: (1) policy level (national or local policy makers); (2) community level (school caterers and their working partners); (3) organisational level (schools); and (4) inter- and intra-personal levels (school/catering staff and children). Data collection methods were then determined by considering their suitability for participants at each socio-ecological level together with their ability to generate data in support of the research aims.

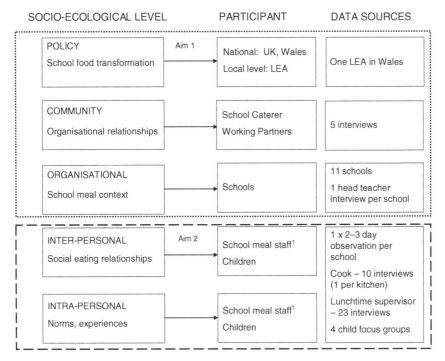

Figure 2. Socio-ecologically informed methods and recruitment strategy.
Note: [1]Catering staff who prepare and serve school meals, together with lunchtime supervisors who support children in the dining hall.

Social ecology as an evaluative framework

Social ecology can further be utilised as an evaluative tool to support data analysis. During the exploratory study into the role of primary school dining halls in improving children's nutrition-related behaviour, a socio-ecological framework was used to evaluate the implementation of school nutritional policies against the policy and needs analysis represented by the theoretical model presented in Figure 1. At the organisational level of analysis, whilst reflecting the primary objective of national policy with respect to the nutritional content of the school meal, LEA and school policies were also influenced by multiple, competing interests including parental views, children's food preferences and organisational objectives such as protecting school meal uptake (Moore *et al.* 2010a). Tensions existed between food availability and choice such that menus incorporating choices based on children's preferences were viewed as facilitating service viability and prioritised over the promotion of healthy eating.

Interactions between the policy, organisational and intra-personal levels were evident in that catering staff were the final arbiters regarding the food actually served to the children since their individual working practices and beliefs influenced the food available (Moore 2011). For example, the menu on offer in a particular school on a particular day not only reflected the various policy decisions that preceded it, but also a range of practical decisions made by the cook-in-charge. These included catering amounts, the selection of 'seasonal' vegetables and the availability of salad accompaniments.

Interactions between the organisational level and inter-personal level were evident with respect to the extent to which children were encouraged to choose menu items by catering staff (Moore *et al.* 2010a). Three different approaches were used: (1) assisting the child to make their choice whilst leaving the final decision with the child; (2) allowing the child freedom of choice; and (3) constraining freedom of choice by mandating what was served. Preferred approaches tended to reflect the personal styles, beliefs and experiences of the catering staff rather than being disseminated in formal policies or training programmes.

With respect to potential reciprocal relationships between pupils and school policy, the format that schools adopted for school council consultations took the form of structured meetings during which the children presented their viewpoints (Moore 2011). These were either solicited from peers using questionnaires or by the researcher/teachers asking specific questions during the council session. Children conceptualised the promotion of healthy eating during school meals in terms of food availability, which was expected to align with personal preferences, as well as food interactions. The latter included being encouraged to eat by school meal staff and the influence of the dining hall context (e.g. the time allocated to eat).

At the intra-organisational level of analysis, the dining halls had numerous generic attributes (e.g. accommodation, equipment, length of lunchtime, social actors) which interacted to have a direct, but not necessarily positive, bearing on food choice and consumption (Moore *et al.* 2010b). For example, for schools with dual purpose dining halls (i.e. used for teaching as well as dining), the times when the hall became available after morning teaching sessions and was then required for afternoon teaching sessions were strictly defined and placed stringent constraints on the time available for eating. Space and the availability of tables and chairs defined each school's seating capacity. When considered in the context of the total number of pupils in the school, no schools could accommodate all pupils (i.e. packed and cooked lunches) in the dining hall at the same time. Overcrowded, multi-purpose dining halls coupled with time pressures and dynamic social situations (e.g. discipline issues) detracted from the eating experience and the ability of staff to encourage children to eat.

At the intra-personal level of analysis, the children's food dislikes featured prominently (Moore *et al.* 2010) and the selection of nutritionally imbalanced meals and/or small portions were frequently observed, despite the best efforts of serving staff. The most common nutrition-related behaviour that serving staff sought to influence was choice, whereas supervisors most commonly sought to influence consumption.

At the inter-personal level of analysis, most feeding strategies used by school meal staff reflected those reported in the literature (e.g. pressure, encouragement and rewards) (Moore *et al.* 2010). Staff readily, if not consistently, used these strategies, although the constraints and opportunities of each dining hall context influenced their selection and implementation. On the other hand, purposeful modelling of nutrition-related behaviours was not found. The imposition of food norms, such as eating dessert last, was common. However, even if children left the service point with nutritionally balanced meals, they were often not fully consumed.

Policy implications

The application of a socio-ecological perspective to explore the role of Welsh primary school dining halls in improving children's nutrition-related behaviour reveals several policy implications. Government policies in the UK have targeted the school meal service as a means of improving nutritional intake and children's nutrition-related behaviour (Evans and Harper 2009). However, the study showed how the food that was actually available for the school meal was dependent on national policy *and* subsequent multi-layered processes whereby organisational and individual experiences and ecologies of practice influenced local implementation. This suggests that the critical role of school meal providers, school cooks, lunchtime supervisors and the children themselves needs to be recognised and strategic partnerships developed to minimise tensions between improved nutritional standards and school meal uptake.

Although UK national policy requires nutritionally balanced school meals to be available (Evans and Harper 2009), it was evident that dislikes for the food on offer, low consumption and poor choices were prevalent amongst the children. Similarly, a number of specific confounds within the school dining hall environment, many of which were articulated by the children themselves, posed a risk to policy objectives. In order to fully exploit the potential of school dining halls to promote healthy eating, greater emphasis on factors such as the eating environment; the time available for eating; the engagement of children in policy decisions; the role of the midday supervisor; and training of school meal staff in the promotion of choice and consumption behaviours is required. In this way, policy and practice could work together to ensure that children *learn* to consume the nutritionally balanced lunches made available to them in the way that the whole school approach advocates.

School meal staff were found to naturally utilise feeding strategies whose effects are well documented in the literature. More rigorous investigation of the effects of *consistently* using such strategies to promote healthy nutrition-related behaviour in school dining halls is recommended. It was also common for schools/staff to impose a norm that an entrée must be eaten before a dessert. As other non-directed behavioural practices were also evident (e.g. queuing, seating), children in school dining halls may readily accept and comply with school-imposed norms to such an extent that the phenomenon could be used to positive effect with respect to further influencing nutrition-related behaviour. Interventions designed to promote the active, ongoing management of children's nutrition-related behaviour by school meal staff have the potential to add synergy to the UK's food transformation programmes.

Conclusion

Socio-ecological models are posited as frameworks for identifying health improvement leverage points and analysing health improvement initiatives (McLeroy *et al.* 1988). By considering the specific example of the role of school dining halls in improving children's nutrition-related behaviour, it has been shown how the application of a socio-ecological perspective facilitated: (1) a theoretical understanding of some of the relationships and process involved, and potential directions for future research; (2) the definition of the methodological approach, methods and recruitment strategy; and (3) the evaluation of policy implementations. Overall, the approach elicited numerous multi-faceted policy implications and associated opportunities to strengthen the socio-ecological reciprocity between policy and behaviour. The latter took the form of policies that emphasise improvements to children's nutrition-related behaviours and the dining hall context *as well as* the nutritional content of school meals. Such policies could contribute to the wider public health agenda through the realisation of positive health-related outcomes associated with improved nutrition-related behaviour. Such outcomes include improvements to long-term health and obesity prevention, and a reduction in health inequalities through the utilisation of the school as a setting which embraces all social classes.

On a more generic level, it is suggested that higher level policy interventions may be limited in their effectiveness if they are undermined by a lack of attention to lower level factors that may compromise their successful implementation. In mitigation, the use of a socio-ecological framework as a theoretical, methodological and evaluative tool capable of supporting a consistent, holistic approach during the design, implementation and evaluation of health improvement policies is recommended.

Acknowledgements

The authors thank all those who participated in this study and the school administrative staff who assisted in the informed consent process. This study was supported by a PhD studentship awarded by the Economic and Social Research Council.

References

Armstrong, J., *et al.*, 2003. Coexistence of social inequalities in undernutrition and obesity in preschool children: population based cross sectional study. *Archives of Disease in Childhood*, 88, 671–675.

Atkinson, P., Coffey, A., and Delamont, S., 2003. *Key themes in qualitative research – continuities and change*. Walnut Creek, CA: AltaMira Press.

Bere, E., *et al.*, 2006. Outcome and process evaluation of a Norwegian school-randomized fruit and vegetable intervention: fruits and vegetables make the marks (FVMM). *Health Education Research*, 21 (2), 258–267.

Birch, L.L., 1998. Development of food acceptance patterns in the first years of life. *Proceedings of the Nutrition Society*, 57 (4), 617–624.

Birch, L.L. and Marlin, D.W., 1982. I don't like it; I never tried it: effects of exposure on two-year old children's food preferences. *Appetite*, 3 (4), 353–360.

Bronfenbrenner, U., 1979. *The ecology of human development*. London: Harvard University Press.

Bronfenbrenner, U., 1986. Ecology of the familiy as a context for human development: research perspectives. *Developmental Psychology*, 22 (6), 723–742.

Chaudhury, M., *et al.*, 2008. *Health survey for England 2007. Healthy lifestyles:knowledge, attitudes and behaviour*. Vol. 1, London: The Information Centre for Health and Social Care.

Ciriza, E., Perez-Rodrigo, C., and Aranceta, J., 2008. The challenge of promoting fruit and vegetable consumption in the school setting. *A systematic review. Spanish Journal of Community Nutrition*, 14, 6–20.

Coffield, F., *et al.*, 2007. How policy impacts on practice and how practice does not impact on policy. *British Educational Research Journal*, 33 (5), 723–741.

Currie, C., *et al.*, 2008. *Inequalities in young people's health. Health behaviour in school-aged children: international report from the 2005/2006 survey*. Copenhagen: World Health Organisation.

Daniel, P. and Gustafsson, U., 2010. School lunches:children's services of children's spaces?. *Children's Geographies*, 8 (3), 265–274.

Davies, S., 2005. *School meals, markets and quality*. London: UNISON.

Day, M.E., *et al.*, 2008. Action schools! BC – healthy eating. Effects of a whole-school model to modifying eating behaviours of elementary school children. *Canadian Journal of Public Health*, 99 (4), 328–331.

de Sa, J. and Lock, K., 2008. Will European agricultural policy for school fruit and vegetables improve public health? A review of school fruit and vegetable programmes. *European Journal of Public Health*, 18 (6), 558–568.

Department of Health, 2005. *Choosing a better diet: a food and health action plan* [online]. Available from: http://www.dh.gov.uk/prod_consum_dh/groups/dh_digitalassets/@dh/@en/documents/digitalasset/dh_4105709.pdf [Accessed 8 April 2010].

Deshmukh-Taskar, P., *et al.*, 2006. Tracking of overweight status from childhood to young adulthood: the Bogalusa Heart Study. *European Journal of Clinical Nutrition*, 60 (1), 48–57.

Dworetzky, J.P., 1995. *Human development. A lifespan approach*. 2nd ed. New York, NY: West.

Evans, C.E.L. and Harper, C.E., 2009. A history and review of school meal standards in the UK. *Journal of Human Nutrition and Dietetics*, 22 (2), 89–99.

Fisher, J.O. and Birch, L.L., 1999. Restricting access to foods and children's eating. *Appetite*, 32 (3), 405–419.

Fisher, J.O., *et al.*, 2002. Parental Influences on young girls' fruit and vegetable, micronutrient and fat intakes. *Journal of the American Dietetic Association*, 102 (1), 58–64.

Food Standards Agency and Department of Health, 2010. *National diet and nutrition survey. Report – headline results from year 1 of the rolling programme (2008/2009)* [online]. Available from: http://www.food.gov.uk/multimedia/pdfs/publication/ndnsreport0809year1results.pdf [Accessed 26 April 2010].

Food Standards Agency Wales, 2003. *Food and well being* [online]. Available from: http://www.food.gov.uk/multimedia/pdfs/foodandwellbeing.pdf [Accessed 4 December 2008].

Foster, P., 1996. *Observing schools. A methodological guide*. London: Paul Chapman.

Gatenby, L.A., 2007. Nutritional content of school meals in Hull and the East Riding of Yorkshire: a comparison of two schools. *Journal of Human Nutrition and Dietetics*, 20 (6), 538–548.

Gould, R., Russell, J., and Barker, M.E., 2006. School lunch menus and 11 to 12 year old children's food choice in three secondary schools in England – are the nutritional standards being met?. *Appetite*, 46 (1), 86–92.

Grzywacz, J.G. and Fuqua, J., 2000. The social ecology of health: leverage points and linkages. *Behavioral medicine*, 26 (3), 101–115.

Health Education Board for Scotland, *et al.*, 1996. The European network of health promoting schools: introduction – the UK project. *Health Education Journal*, 55 (4), 447–449.

Hendy, H.M. and Raudenbush, B., 2000. Effectiveness of teacher modelling to encourage food acceptance in preschool children. *Appetite*, 34 (1), 61–76.

Hendy, H.M., Williams, K.E., and Camise, T.S., 2005. Kids choice school lunch program increases children's fruit and vegetable acceptance. *Appetite*, 45 (3), 250–263.

Horne, P.J., *et al.*, 2004. Increasing children's fruit and vegetable consumption: a peer modelling and rewards-based intervention. *European Journal of Clinical Nutrition*, 58 (12), 1649–1660.

Kelder, S.H., *et al.*, 1994. Longitudinal tracking of adolescent smoking, physical activity and food choice behaviours. *American Journal of Public Health*, 84 (7), 1121–1126.

Learning and Teaching Scotland, 2009. *Curriculum for excellence: food and health* [online]. Available from: http://www.ltscotland.org.uk/curriculumforexcellence/healthandwellbeing/outcomes/foodandhealth/index.asp [Accessed 23 September 2009].

Lister-Sharp, D., *et al.*, 1999. Health promoting schools and health promotion in schools: two systematic reviews. *Health Technology Assessment*, 3 (22), 1–207.

McGee, D.L. and Diverse Populations, Collaboration, 2005. Body mass index and mortality: a meta-analysis based on person-level data from twenty-six observational studies. *Annals of Epidemiology*, 15 (2), 87–97.

McLaren, L. and Hawe, P., 2005. Ecological perspectives in health research. *Journal of Epidemiology and Community Health*, 59, 6–14.

McLeroy, K.R., *et al.*, 1988. An ecological perspective on health promotion programs. *Health Education Quarterly*, 15 (4), 351–377.

Moore, S.N., 2011. *Improving the eating behaviours of primary schoolchildren*. Unpublished doctoral thesis, Cardiff University, Cardiff.

Moore, S.N., *et al.*, 2010a. From policy to plate: barriers to implementing healthy eating policies in primary schools in Wales. *Health Policy*, 94 (3), 239–245.

Moore, S.N., *et al.*, 2010b. The social, physical and temporal characteristics of primary school dining halls and their implications for children's eating behaviours. *Health Education*, 110 (5), 399–411.

Moore, S.N., Tapper, K., and Murphy, S., 2007. Feeding strategies used by mothers of 3-5-year-old children. *Appetite*, 49 (3), 704–707.

Moore, S.N., Tapper, K., and Murphy, S., 2010. Feeding strategies used by primary school meal staff and their impact on children's eating. *Journal of Human Nutrition and Dietetics*, 23 (1), 78–84.

Morgan, K., 2006. School food and the public domain: the politics of the public plate. *The Political Quarterly*, 77 (3), 379–387.

Mukoma, W. and Flisher, A.J., 2004. Evaluations of Health promoting schools: a review of nine studies. *Health Promotion International*, 19 (3), 357–368.

National Institute for Health and Clinical Excellence, 2010. *Public health guidance 25. Prevention of cardiovascular disease at population level* [online]. Available from: http://www.nice.org.uk/nicemedia/live/13024/49273/49273.pdf [Accessed 30 January 2011].

Paisley, C., *et al.*, 2006. *Pupils' food choices and the factors influencing choice in primary and secondary schools in Wales*. Bangor: Bangor University.

Parsons, C., Stears, D., and Thomas, C., 1996. The health promoting school in Europe: conceptualising and evaluating the change. *Health Education Journal*, 55 (3), 311–321.

Piaget, J. and Inhelder, B., 1969. *The psychology of the child*. London: Routledge and Kegan Paul.

Pike, J., 2008. Foucault, space and primary school dining rooms. *Children's Geographies*, 6 (4), 413–422.

Pike, J., 2010. I don't have to listen to you! You're just a dinner lady!: power and resistance at lunchtimes in primary schools. *Children's Geographies*, 8 (3), 275–287.

Pike, J. and Colquhoun, D., 2009. The relationship between policy and place:the role of school meals in addressing health inequalities. *Health Sociology Review*, 18 (1), 50–60.

Rasmussen, M., *et al.*, 2006. Determinants of fruit and vegetable consumption among children and adolescents:a review of the literature. *Part 1: quantitative. International Journal of Behavioral Nutrition and Physical Activity*, 3 (1), 22.

Resnicow, K., *et al.*, 1997. Social-cognitive predictors of fruit and vegetable intake in children. *Health Psychology*, 16 (3), 272–276.

School Food Trust, 2007. *A fresh look at the school meal experience* [online]. Available from: http://www.schoolfoodtrust.org.uk/doc_item.asp?DocId=45andDocCatId=9 [Accessed 6 April 2009].

School Meals Review Panel, 2005. *Turning the tables: transforming school food* [online]. Available from: http://www.dfes.gov.uk/consultations/downloadableDocs/SMRP%20Report%20FINAL.pdf [Accessed 19 January 2007].

Schwartz, M.B., 2007. The influence of a verbal prompt on school lunch fruit consumption: a pilot study. *International Journal of Behavioral Nutrition and Physical Activity*, 4, 6.

Scottish Executive, 2002. *Hungry for success – a whole school approach to school meals in Scotland* [online]. Available from: http://www.scotland.gov.uk/Resource/Doc/47032/0023961.pdf [Accessed 18 January 2007].

Scottish Executive, 2004. *Eating for health: meeting the challenge* [online]. Available from: http://www.scotland.gov.uk/Publications/2004/07/19624/39995 [Accessed 8 April 2010].

Stamatakis, E., Wardle, J., and Cole, T.J., 2010. Childhood obesity and overweight prevalence trends in England: evidence for growing socioeconomic disparities. *International Journal of Obesity*, 34 (1), 41–47.

Stark, L.J., *et al.*, 1986. Using reinforcement and cueing to increase healthy snack food choices in preschoolers. *Journal of Applied Behavior Analysis*, 19 (4), 367–379.

Stokols, D., 1992. Establishing and maintaining healthy environments. *American Psychologist*, 47 (1), 6–22.

Stroebele, N. and De Castro, J.M., 2004. Effect of ambience on food intake and food choice. *Nutrition*, 20 (9), 821–838.

Stronach, I., *et al.*, 2002. Towards an uncertain politics of professionalism: teacher and nurse identities in flux. *Journal of Educational Policy*, 7 (1), 110–138.

The Health and Social Care Information Centre, 2010. *Health survey for England 2009. Volume 1: health and lifestyles* [online]. Available from: http://www.ic.nhs.uk/webfiles/publications/003_Health_Lifestyles/hse09report/HSE_09_Volume1.pdf [Accessed 5 February 2011].

The Scottish Government, 2010. *Scottish Health Survey 2009 – Volume 1: Main report* [online]. Available from: http://www.scotland.gov.uk/Publications/2010/09/23154223/0 [Accessed 3 February 2011].

US Department of Agriculture, 2011. *Nutrition standards in the national school lunch and school breakfast programs: proposed rule* [online]. Available from: http://www.fns.usda.gov/cnd/Governance/regulations/2011-01-13.pdf [Accessed 10 May 2011].

Wardle, J., 2005. Understanding the aetiology of childhood obesity: implications for treatment. *Proceedings of the Nutrition Society*, 64 (1), 73–79.

Welsh Government, 2008a. *Appetite for life action plan* [online]. Available from: http://wales.gov.uk/docs/dcells/publications/091207appetiteforlifeen.pdf [Accessed 2 August 2010].

Welsh Government, 2008b. *Learning across the curriculum. Personal and social education.* Cardiff: Welsh Government.

Welsh Government, 2010. *Appetite for life action research project 2008–2010* [online]. Available from: http://wales.gov.uk/docs/caecd/research/101216appetiteforlifeen.doc#_Toc276738165 [Accessed 27 January 2011].

World Cancer Research Fund, 2007. *SUMMARY Food, nutrition, physical activity and the prevention of cancer: a global perspective* [online]. Available from: http://www.dietand-cancerreport.org/downloads/summary/english.pdf [Accessed 30 January 2011].

World Health Organisation, 1986. *The Ottawa charter for health promotion.* Copenhagen: WHO.

World Health Organisation, 1991. *Sundsvall statement on supportive environments for health. Report from the third international conference on health promotion*, 9–15 June 1991. Sundsvall, Sweden. Copenhagen: WHO.

World Health Organisation, 1997. *Jakarta declaration on leading health promotion into the 21st century* [online]. Available from: http://www.who.int/healthpromotion/conferences/previous/jakarta/declaration/en/index.html [Accessed 16 April 2010].

World Health Organisation, 2003. *Diet, nutrition and the prevention of chronic diseases. report of a joint WHO/FAO expert consultation. WHO technical report series. 916* [online]. Available from: http://whqlibdoc.who.int/trs/WHO_TRS_916.pdf [Accessed 14 April 2010].

World Health Organisation, 2009. *What is a health promoting school* [online]. Available from: http://www.who.int/school_youth_health/gshi/hps/en/ [Accessed 23 September 2009].

Food insecurity in South Australian single parents: an assessment of the livelihoods framework approach

Iain R. Law[a], Paul R. Ward[b] and John Coveney[b]

[a]School of Medicine, Flinders University, Adelaide, Australia; [b]Discipline of Public Health, Flinders University, Adelaide, Australia

Single parent households experience periods of food insecurity more frequently than other Australian families. Despite elevated risk, many single parents achieve food security with limited means. This article applies and evaluates the utility of the livelihoods framework approach as a tool for understanding food insecurity in this population and generating relevant policy recommendations. The approach is adapted here to provide insight into the skills, strategies and resource individuals use to attain or strive for food security. The framework incorporates these individual capabilities into a model of the social, economic and political structures and processes through which individuals navigate to attain food security. Semi-structured interviews were conducted with single parents living in rural and urban South Australia. Transcripts were analysed in an effort to populate a food security livelihoods framework for single parents. The livelihoods framework is found to be capable of reproducing the types and levels of capabilities reported in previous findings. Furthermore, it provides novel insight into the relationships that form between classes of capabilities and between capabilities and the structures and processes in which they are utilised. These insights are considered in terms of relevance to policy.

Introduction

In a document entitled *Australia: The Healthiest Country by 2020*, released in June 2009, the National Preventative Health Taskforce (NPHT) described obesity as one of three priority action areas for better health, besides tobacco and alcohol consumption. It emphasised that addressing social inequalities in differential access to healthy food is fundamental to obesity prevention (National Preventative Health Taskforce 2009). In doing so, the NPHT identified food insecurity as an important concern for low-income Australians and many at-risk groups, and acknowledged the ensuing negative health consequences of inadequate access to healthy food. This article investigates determinants of food insecurity experienced by one such at-risk group; low-income single parents in South Australia.

Effective policy needs to respond to a wide array of determinants. The Department for International Development (1999) in the UK formulated the livelihoods framework approach for guiding policy in developing countries. The approach is adapted here to provide insight into the skills, strategies and resource individuals use to attain or strive for food security. The framework incorporates these individual capabilities into a model of the social, economic and political structures and processes through which individuals navigate to attain food security. At time of writing, the livelihoods framework approach has not been applied to the problem of food insecurity in developed countries. In an effort to explore and evaluate the opportunities provided by this approach, we apply it to the lived experiences of single parents in South Australia.

Food security, within developed countries such as Australia, can be defined as, the 'ability of individuals, households and communities to acquire appropriate and nutritious food on a regular and reliable basis, and using socially acceptable means' (Rychetnik *et al.* 2003, p. 1). The 1995 National Nutrition Survey estimates food insecurity in Australia at 5.2% in the general population (Marks *et al.* 2001). Data collected in South Australia estimate the food insecurity rate to be approximately 7% (Foley *et al.* 2010). However, this increases among at-risk groups including: unemployed (11.3%), rental households (15.8%) (Marks *et al.* 2001), those identifying as Aboriginal or Torres Strait Islander (23%) (Shannon 2002) and recently landed refugees (71%) (Gallegos *et al.* 2008). Single parents are also considered an at-risk group with reported levels of food insecurity as high as 23% (Burns 2004).

The health consequences of food insecurity are well documented. It might be expected that food insecurity would be associated with reduced food intake and below average body mass. However, in a developed country, food insecurity is associated with obesity (Alaimo *et al.* 2001b, Townsend *et al.* 2001, Burns 2004, Martin and Ferris 2007) and obesity-related disease (Vozoris and Tarasuk 2003, Seligman *et al.* 2007). These elevated rates of obesity among the food insecure is thought to result principally from increased consumption of foods high in fat and or sugar that are typically cheaper, more available, heavily marketed and simpler to prepare than healthy alternatives (Burns 2004, Drewnowski and Specter 2004, Wong *et al.* 2011). Furthermore, the health consequences of food insecurity go beyond obesity and include nutrient inadequacy (Kirkpatrick and Tarasuk 2008), poor self-reported health (Vozoris and Tarasuk 2003) and compromised child health (Alaimo *et al.* 2001a).

Diverse factors differentially expose certain members of the population to periods of food insecurity and the associated consequences. Some established determinants include: poverty (Polit *et al.* 2000), rising food prices in Australia (Harrison *et al.* 2007), higher food prices and greater density of unhealthy food options in socially disadvantaged areas (Donkin *et al.* 2000, Ellaway and Macintyre 2000), other financial obligations (Kirkpatrick and Tarasuk 2007), employment status (McIntyre 2003), lower educational attainment (Turrell and Kavanagh 2006) and lack of access to private transport (Coveney and O'Dwyer 2009).

Single parents experience an elevated risk of food insecurity due to increased poverty rates compared to partnered families (Gucciardi *et al.* 2004, Page and Stevens 2004, Glanville and McIntyre 2006). There is also a tendency for single parents to sacrifice their own nutrition to improve the diet of their children (Dowler 1997, McIntyre *et al.* 2003a). The lived experience of low-income single parents is characterised by feeling deprived, frustrated by a lack of occupational choice, needing to manage the appearance of poverty, judged and degraded by other families, guilt in relation to their children and isolated from social activities (McIntyre *et al.* 2003b). These findings are of increasing concern as the Australian Bureau of Statistics reports that the number of single parents continues to climb (Australian Bureau of Statistics 2007).

In this article, we apply the livelihoods framework approach as an analytical lens and organisational structure and is expected to generate policy relevant understanding of the strategies single parents use to maintain food security, the limits of those strategies and the socioeconomic environment in which these strategies emerge. The utility of the framework is evaluated in terms of the consistency of its findings to previous literature and the novel insight it provides and compared with other candidate frameworks to provide critical insight into potential limitations.

Methods

Theoretical framework

The livelihoods framework is adapted from the Department for International Development (1999) and Women and Economic Development Consortium (2001). It is an assets, as opposed to deficits, model (Sen 1999) that depicts the main factors that impact an individual's capacity to maintain a sustainable livelihood (Figure 1). Sustainable livelihood refers to the life situation that people strive towards that enables individuals to, 'maintain and cultivate ourselves and our households, to take advantage of opportunities for growth over time and to remain resistant to shocks and stresses from within and without' (Department for International Development 1999, p. 12). The extent to which someone is able to achieve a sustainable livelihood is a function of the first three components of the framework: (1) vulnerability context, (2) livelihood capabilities and (3) transforming structures and processes. These components do not interact in a linear fashion. Rather, they relate to one another dynamically with influence travelling in all directions. Through these components, the framework captures both individual and structural determinants of achieving a sustainable livelihood.

The vulnerability context comprises the physical, social, political and economic environments in which people live and shapes and constrains capacity to achieve sustainable livelihoods. The other components of the model respond to the

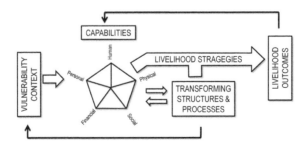

Figure 1. The livelihoods framework. Adapted from Department for International Development (1999) and Serrat (2010).

vulnerability context. Capabilities represent fluid and exchangeable personal assets and attributes utilised to achieve livelihoods. The five capabilities are: (1) physical, (2) human, (3) financial, (4) social and (5) personal.

Physical capabilities include the natural resources, equipment, services and infrastructure available to a person. In terms of food insecurity, this includes access to, and availability of, healthy food. Human capabilities reflect the health, skills and knowledge that allow someone to earn money and apply other capabilities to their maximum effectiveness. Financial capabilities are the financial resources a person has available and generally come from two main sources: savings, or other liquid assets, and regular income. Social capabilities are the social and political networks to which someone belongs that can be utilised to achieve a sustainable livelihood. Personal capabilities stem from values and self-perceptions. These drive motivation and enable personal transformation.

Finally, the transforming structures and processes reflect the institutions, organisations, policies, social structures, cultures, markets and laws through which people utilise their capabilities to produce sustainable livelihoods. Although they do not directly affect capabilities, the livelihood outcomes they engender feedback and allow individuals to invest in the capabilities they need for a sustainable future.

Data collection

The research took a qualitative, inductive approach. This enabled interviewers to draw out the world-views of the participants and limited the influence of researchers' preconceptions of either the relative importance of food security or the factors that lead to participants being food insecure. Participants were not predetermined as 'food insecure', but rather interviewers provided space for them to talk freely about all issues to do with accessing, cooking and storing food.

A semi-structured interview was used, which allowed for explorations and discussions of relevant experiences and perceptions of history, biography and food, in addition to creating an atmosphere conducive to an open and uninhibited flow of conversation (Silverman 2001). In this way, the interview process and later data analysis recognised that 'food security' may not have been a useful concept to understand food-related behaviours within these particular groups.

In total, 73 interviews were undertaken, although this particular article focuses on single parent families, which was a subset of 8 interviews (Table 1). The project was approved by the Social and Behavioural Research Ethics Committee (Project Number 4415). Informed consent was obtained before all interviews. A stratified sample (SES, household type and geographic location) was recruited by Harrison's, an accredited social research agency. This approach to sampling has been successfully used by the research team before, and is particularly useful for accessing 'hard to reach' groups, such as single parent families.

Interviews were undertaken with all willing participants within each household and explored the opportunities and barriers to access food outlets and healthy food choices. The interview covered areas such as regular food shopping destinations, reasons for food choice and value for money and perceptions on the influence of food advertising on purchasing habits.

Interviews generally lasted 1 h, were undertaken at a venue convenient to the participant and were all audio-recorded and transcribed verbatim.

Table 1. Respondent demographics.

Respondent	Age	Gender	Number of children	Highest level of education	Employment
R1	34	F	1	Year 12	Disability
R2	48	F	2	Year 12	Casual part time
R3	27	F	3	Year 11	Pension
R4	27	F	1	Year 12	Casual part time
R5	53	M	1	Year 10	Disability
R6	44	F	4	Advanced Diploma	Permanent part time, Pension
R7	54	F	1	BSc	Permanent part time
R8	25	F	1	Advanced Diploma	Permanent part time, Pension

Notes: 'Disability' refers to income support for persons who suffer from a long-term disability. 'Pension' refers to income support available to single parents in need.

Preliminary analysis, with recording of field notes, was carried out soon after each interview in order to inform the development of subsequent interviews. All transcripts were checked for accuracy by a member of the research team. Initial analysis of all 73 transcripts involved open coding, and then grouping conceptual labels under common themes which were modified to accommodate negative or deviant findings. Through the analytic process, it became clearer which themes were common, not only across the study participants, but within sub-groups as well (e.g. single parents, older participants, rural/metro participants, etc). It became clear that single parents had particular issues in relation to accessing food which were not common to other participants in the study and deserved independent consideration. These issues emerge from the lifestyle demands of supporting children alone including, extensive demands on time, resources spent on childcare, restricted income and the challenges of balancing work, necessities of daily living and parenting.

Analytical process

In terms of analysis for this article, the objective was to populate a food insecurity livelihoods framework for low-income single parents. The livelihoods framework functioned as an analytic lens through which the data were viewed and organised. To accommodate this function, the 'framework method' (Ritchie and Spencer 1994) of analysis was adopted to replace open coding. The framework method facilitates qualitative analysis that is directed a priori by a specific research objective, but remains responsive to emergent themes within the data or as identified by respondents themselves. In contrast to the initial analysis of all transcripts, components of the livelihoods framework constituted thematic nodes and provided thematic hierarchy. Each interview transcript was coded and indexed according to components of the livelihoods framework, including vulnerability context, each type of capability and transforming structures and processes. Sections of text referring to a particular livelihoods framework component were copied to their appropriate node. This facilitated interpretation of each component across respondents. Portions of interviews found to be incompatible with the livelihoods framework were indexed and analysed according to their internal emergent themes.

Findings

Analysis of the interview data enabled the construction of a food insecurity livelihoods framework for the single parent sample. However, two caveats must be considered. First, the intention was to understand the experience of the respondents. Therefore, the focus was on what impedes these parents from achieving their expectation of a healthy diet, rather than determining the disparity between their diets and a clinical definition of a healthy diet. Second, this was a secondary use of data in that the interview was not specifically designed to elicit information pertinent to a livelihoods framework approach. As a result, some sections may be disproportionately populated. Also, the dataset only included eight single parent respondents, which diminishes the comprehensiveness of the findings. Although these data proved sufficient to populate a preliminary livelihoods framework useful for evaluating this approach, our findings relating to food insecurity for single parents are tentative and subject to confirmation through further investigation.

Vulnerability context

Respondents' discussion of issues pertinent to the vulnerability context was limited, likely due to the content of the interview questions. Issues discussed included: increasing price of food over time and of fruit and vegetables in particular; shrinking package sizes while maintaining prices; and diminishing food quality, especially of fruit and vegetables. The demands of single parenthood, including managing children while shopping, children's dietary restrictions and preferences and meeting the needs of multiple children and their friends were also reported.

Financial capabilities

The financial capabilities of respondents varied from full-time employment to pensioners, those on permanent disability cover and those on welfare. Respondents consistently reported income as the dominant, and usually the only factor that limits food purchases, indicating a relative deprivation of financial capabilities within this group:

> The last two weeks I actually put myself on a budget, so I bought just the basics of what I needed. [R4]
>
> Like I think I need to have more in the area of fruit. We don't eat nearly as much fruit, but I can't afford the bloody fruit. [R5]
>
> Obviously, if I had unlimited spending power I would buy a lot more, but I buy enough to suit my family. [R6]

Notably, these restrictions were most acute for central food items such as fruits, vegetables and meat. However, as strained as financial capabilities appear to be, the respondents maintain that they are able to provide for their families.

Social capabilities

Respondents commonly reported two types of social capabilities. First were exchange relationships, where friends or family brought food around. This was usually eggs (it is not unusual in South Australia for homes to keep one or more chickens for egg laying purposes), but fruit and vegetables, or a hamper, were also reported. A second relevant social capability is amicable relations with shop owners, or employees of supermarkets, which benefit respondents in terms of what food is made available and what they pay for it.

> I go to Foodland [large supermarket chain] and get it from there because I know the lady that works there and she tells me which ones are the cheapest. [R3]

> You know, if you wanted to buy a cow [from the butcher] you'd have to start talking to the butchers and find out what their intent is otherwise you're bidding against them and you can't bid against the butchers. [R5]

Personal capabilities

Data relevant to personal capabilities were limited. Respondents discussed pride in thriftiness and the value they place on providing healthy and nutritious food for their families.

> I bargain hunt. I'm a champion bargain hunter. [R2]

> Well you've got to live within your means....but food is one thing I will not scrimp out on. If it means I can't go to the gym or, you know, I can't go out or anything I won't. [R8]

> I won't go without food, no. I mean I can live on beans on toast or spaghetti on toast, but [my child] can't so you can't skimp on food. [R8]

Physical capabilities

Some physical capabilities were relatively consistent across respondents. Almost all used a car to transport groceries. Supermarkets were the dominant source of groceries and all respondents, even those in rural locations, lived less than 5 kilometres from a large supermarket. No respondent indicated they had trouble accessing food.

Other, more variable, physical capabilities that contribute to food security were gardens and storage space. Some respondents had home gardens and fruit trees, but these appeared to contribute minimally to diet. Storage and freezer space was generally good, and a crucial asset to many parents who depend upon saving money by buying in bulk and freezing meals to reduce cost and waste.

Human capabilities

Respondents exhibit extensive and various human capabilities that enable them to achieve food security. A major contributor was knowledge and skills that enable good purchasing decisions, including bargain hunting, evaluating 'specials' [offers] and knowing stores in the area:

> They send out a catalogue every week and I cruise the shops. Well they can't fit everything in the catalogue that's on special. [R2]

> I'll have a look 'okay, that's meant to be on special, I'll go down the aisle and see if there's anything similar to that' [R3]

I did have to look around because I did feel, because of the lack of department stores, that things were more expensive. Now I've got to know all the different stores I know which items I can get that are similar at a cheaper price. [R6]

Other contributing human capabilities included: competency at cooking and related strategies such as batch cooking and freezing:

[It's] about having the knowledge and knowing what to buy and then once you've bought it knowing what to do with it. [R5]

I mean I'm a cooker so I will use something for a base and just add whatever I want to it so I don't mind going for the cheaper option. [R8]

Health knowledge about the importance of fruits and vegetables and eating a balanced diet was also reported. However, in other areas, there was a relative deprivation of human capabilities. For example, health was an issue for many respondents. It impeded their ability to shop, lift large or bulk items and restricted what they could eat.

Time capabilities

During the analysis, it became apparent that some respondents were constrained by the amount of time they had in the day to accomplish everything, including food acquisition and preparation.

It's terrible when you work – I've been working full-time and doing all sorts of other things, that's why I go in my lunch hour. And you've got to get back on time. I've got one hour from when I leave work until I have to get back so, yes. [R7]

Oh sometimes I skip lunch just because I'm busy. [R6]

like Wednesday nights for us is busy, she has school then she comes – goes to swimming and then to her grandma's for piano lessons so it's always good just to [have a meal] out of the freezer... [R1]

Time was most constraining for working parents and less so for those on pensions or disability.

Transforming structures and processes

Respondents identified a variety of structures and processes, such as social services, the educational system and cultural norms that influence food security. However, supermarkets – the dominant food source for this group – emerged as a crucial structure and process for transforming capabilities into livelihoods.

Respondent engagement with supermarkets is complex. Parents rely on promotions offered by supermarkets to stay within their food budgets, which fosters an impression of generosity in some respondents:

And I guess I buy according to specials...Sometimes I don't buy it because it's too expensive, so you go without, especially meat. I won't buy it usually full price so you've got to wait for the specials. That's very limiting. [R7]

Coles is trying to be better for people. At the moment they've got their watermelon out for 96 cents a kilo which is better than paying two dollars a kilo. [R1]

In situations where specials are unavailable or sold out, frustrations are sometimes directed towards other customers:

It's hard to do it sometimes because some people get here really, really early and all the specials have all gone and like why can't people just have variety and have the different one which is also on special but they don't like it because it's got such and such on it. I'm like 'come on'. [R3]

However, respondents also acknowledge the limits of promotions to meet their dietary needs:

R: But, meat does go on special frequently, but not much in the store does. They have a lot of specials on chocolates and drinks and things, soft drinks, but they don't have the specials on <inaudible>.
I: The stuff you really need which is...
R: So they don't have that kind of stuff. [R1]

Furthermore, respondents report the capacity for supermarkets to be deceitful. This is apparent in comments reported in the vulnerability context and human capabilities section regarding the shrinking of packages and their contents without a corresponding reduction in price and the need to double check the value of specials. Other supermarket tactics are also questioned by respondents:

When that GST [(Government Sales Tax] stuff was all getting talked about I noticed that from that day on every couple of weeks Woolworth was putting the prices up, not to worry about oh, you know, you're getting 10 percent – that's all it is, 10 percent – that's not true. Woolworths had already put the bloomin' price up 10 percent before the GST even got here so the foodstuffs went up 20 or 30 percent. [R5]

In summary, respondents described a complex and contradictory relationship with supermarkets, characterised by dependency, impressions of generosity and recognition of deceit. The implications of this relationship are taken up later in the discussion.

Discussion

We have used the livelihoods framework as both an analytical lens through which qualitative data can be analysed and an organisational structure to model the determinants of food insecurity for low-income single parents in South Australia. We now evaluate utility of this approach, first in terms of the kinds and levels of capabilities it detected compared with previous findings, and second, in terms of novel contribution. Specific contributions discussed include: (1) the dynamic interaction of capabilities and (2) the interaction between capabilities and transforming structures and processes. Finally, the limitations and applications of the livelihoods framework are discussed.

Assessment of capabilities

Capabilities are an inventory of assets or attributes that parents use to achieve food security. Consistent with previous findings, respondents reported a relative deprivation of financial capabilities, mainly in terms of income (Tarasuk 2001, Vozoris and Tarasuk 2003, Glanville and McIntyre 2006, Tarasuk and Vogt 2009, Stevens 2010).

Also consistent with the literature, human capabilities such as cooking skill and storage techniques (McLaughlin *et al.* 2003, Stevens 2010), budget shopping and meal planning (Dowler 1997, Stevens 2010) were found to contribute significantly to food security.

Reports of personal capabilities were limited in our study, which may be due to us analysing secondary data (i.e. the original study was not focussed on capabilities and therefore did not seek to elicit data on personal capabilities). However, capabilities that were identified, including pride in thriftiness and value placed on healthy eating are consistent with the literature (Crotty *et al.* 1992, McIntyre *et al.* 2003b, Burns 2004).

Physical capabilities identified also corroborated previous findings. Consistent with Coveney and O'Dwyer (2009), supermarkets were the principal food source and other sources contributed variably to food security. All respondents reported adequate geographical access to supermarkets and depended on cars for transport.

In terms of social capabilities, there is evidence for people utilizing relationships with family and friends for free food (McIntyre *et al.* 2002). Beyond these exchange relationship, some respondents also discussed the benefits of a relationship with shop or supermarket employees. However, this appears only as a contributory and not a major determinant for achieving food security.

During analyses, it became evident that having sufficient time to complete daily activities was a key issue for these parents. Considering the prevalence of observations, it seems reasonable to incorporate them into the framework. Indeed the importance of time, poverty has been recognised in previous food insecurity research (Drewnowski and Eichelsdoerfer 2009).

Dynamics of capabilities

The preceding discussion demonstrates that the capabilities detected by a livelihoods framework approach are consistent with previous findings. A major strength of this approach is the organization and integration of various determinants of food insecurity. In terms of capabilities themselves, the framework demonstrates that parents reported in this study have developed a wide range of human and social capabilities to substitute for variable deprivation of financial and time capabilities. This form of intra-capability exchange reflects what Department for International Development (1999) identifies as substitution. Bargain hunting reduces food costs. Cooking skill allows parents to buy cheaper unprepared food items. Knowing the layout of the store reduces shopping time. Extensive planning and scheduling allows for food shopping and preparation to be included in a busy day. Relationships with store owners and employees ensure good value for money. The organization provided by the livelihoods framework analysis suggests that although few of these families were currently experiencing food insecurity, the extent of capability substitution suggests their capacity to handle shifts in vulnerability context is compromised.

Capabilities and transforming structures and processes

Another major strength of the framework emerges from the insight it provides into the interaction between individual capabilities and transforming structures and processes. Modelling this interaction reveals the purpose and action of capabilities and the factors that shape, enable, and constrain, ++ their usefulness.

In this study, supermarkets were identified as playing a major transformative role. Structurally, supermarkets are important because their extensive distribution provides geographical access to food. Supermarkets also generate the process, or 'rules of the game', through which respondents access food. This process engenders a complex relationship with supermarkets characterised by dependency, and perceptions of both generosity and deceit. The dependency on promotions appears to foster a willingness to characterise supermarkets as generous and benevolent that disempowers respondents from challenging supermarket processes and protects supermarket from critique. This is apparent, for example, in the frustrated comments directed towards other customers when specials are sold out. However, supermarkets were not immune to criticism by respondents and some deceitful practices were still reported.

The structure and process of supermarkets also characterise the capabilities described by respondents. For example, as described in the findings, cars are commonly used to transport large quantities of groceries, purchasing knowledge and skills catered to bargain hunting and price comparison, and in one case, a relationship was developed with a supermarket employee.

This analysis confirms the importance of supermarkets for these families to maintain food security. As an assets rather than a deficits model, the livelihoods framework approach directs policy makers towards interventions that empower individuals. In this case, policy might engage with supermarket processes to enhance the opportunities for individuals to utilise their existing capabilities. As a commercial enterprise, supermarkets are accountable only to their shareholders. However, revised public policy could focus on increasing accountability to communities through increased transparency of food pricing structures, profit margins and promotional schemes. This could also include taxing unhealthy foods and subsidising healthy foods or regulatory policies such as price controls. Importantly, the model emphasises that attaining sustainable livelihoods feeds back on existing capabilities to strengthen individuals and their communities. These policy approaches are consistent with recommendation that food policy needs to focus upstream on the food supply chain (Caraher and Coveney 2004, Wardle and Baranovic 2009).

The policy relevant evidence produced by the livelihoods framework could have direct implications for national policy in Australia. The National Preventative Health Strategy (NPHS) has made recommendations consistent with the findings of this study. For example, action 2.2 recommends the government should '[c]ommission a review of economic policies and taxation systems, and develop methods for using taxation, grants, pricing, incentives and/or subsidies....' (National Preventative Health Taskforce 2009, p. 105). Unfortunately, in response to the NPHS, the government reported that it had already undertaken a review of the Australian taxation system and that no such policy changes were recommended (Commonwealth of Australia 2010). The NPHS did not make any recommendations for increased transparency and regulation of pricing structures and promotional strategies. The limited scope of the NPHS and the reluctance of the government to engage with structural determinants is unfortunate as policies that engage with transforming structures and processes have potential to improve the livelihood outcomes, which in turn empowers individuals to invest in capabilities needed to achieve their own food security (Department for International Development 1999).

Limitations of the livelihoods framework

The livelihoods framework is an effective policy tool. However, it is not without limitation. A notable issue is the tendency of the framework to treat people as being driven primarily by necessity and ignoring the rich socio-cultural context that motivates certain behaviours. That is to say, the livelihoods framework does not take account of the ways in which people interact with each other and with the cultural environment in which they operate. In an effort to moderate such structuralist accounts of human behaviour, some researchers have turned to Bourdieu (1984) to integrate structure and individual agency (Gatrell *et al.* 2004, Sayer 2005, Lunnay *et al.* 2011). Bourdieu's concepts of 'capital' and 'habitus' might provide similar insight if applied to the livelihoods framework.

Bourdieu's 'capitals' are already reflected in, and behave similarly to, livelihoods framework capabilities and include economic, cultural, social and symbolic capitals. The first three find analogues in financial, human and social capabilities, respectively. However, symbolic capital reflecting prestige, status and authority is missing from the livelihoods framework. Its inclusion would begin to facilitate a richer interpretation of food-related behaviour. For example, it may inform us about why some parents bought organic, or why some choose the premium cheese.

The concept of habitus is particularly useful to mediate between the social structures that constrain behaviour, what Bourdieu refers to as the 'field', and the agency of individuals (Shilling 1993). Habitus reflects a person's 'world-view' (Gatrell *et al.* 2004), or what Bourdieu and Wacquant (1992) describe as the, 'mental and corporeal schemata of perception, appreciation, and action' (p. 16). It suggests that while the social environments, or fields, we experience, are structured and constraining, habitus guides each person's unique navigation of these fields. A popular analogy is the football player who does what he wants on the pitch, but is constrained by the rules of the game.

The livelihoods framework does acknowledge 'culture' as a transforming structure and process, which could be interpreted as reflecting habitus. However, its peripheral allocation deemphasises individual agency afforded by habitus and arguably disempowers the subject of analysis.

Conclusions

Despite these potential shortcomings, the livelihoods framework approach provides critical insight into the needs and challenges of the food insecure population pertinent to policy intervention. These parents, although not consistently food insecure, were found to be exposed to risk of food insecurity resulting from subtle shifts in vulnerability context. This elevated risk is reflected in the deprivation of financial and time capabilities, accompanied by high levels of capability substitution, as parents endeavour to compensate for that deprivation. The framework illuminated potential spaces for policy intervention, including increased transparency of supermarket pricing schemes and promotions and supporting increased regulation of food markets, through taxation and subsidies as opposed to industry self-regulation.

These insights into the lived experience of these parents and subsequent policy options were made visible through the livelihoods framework functioning as both analytic lens and organizational structure. Researchers and policy makers should consider the livelihoods framework when they encounter social outcomes with complex determinants and when policy makers desire to empower individuals to improve their own circumstances.

Acknowledgements

The authors thank Robert Muller for providing the transcripts to the interviews he conducted and the South Australian Department of Health for funding the study under their Strategic Health Priorities Program.

References

Alaimo, K., Olson, C.M., and Frongillo, E.A., 2001a. Low family income and food insufficiency in relation to overweight in us children: is there a paradox? *Archives of Pediatrics and Adolescent Medicine*, 155 (10), 1161–1167.

Alaimo, K., *et al.*, 2001b. Food insufficiency, family income, and health in us preschool and school-aged children. *American Journal of Public Health*, 91 (5), 781–786.

Australian Bureau of Statistics, 2007. *Yearbook of Australia (cat. No. 1301.0)*. Canberra: Australian Bureau of Statistics.

Bourdieu, P., 1984. *Distinction: a social critique of the judgement of taste*. Cambridge, MA: Harvard University Press.

Bourdieu, P. and Wacquant, I.J.D., 1992. *An invitation to reflexive sociology*. Chicago, IL: University of Chicago Press.

Burns, C., 2004. *A review of the literature describing the link between poverty, food insecurity and obesity with specific reference to Australia*. Melbourne: Vichealth.

Caraher, M. and Coveney, J., 2004. Public health nutrition and food policy. *Public Health Nutrition*, 7 (5), 591–598.

Commonwealth of Australia, 2010. *Taking preventative action – a response to Australia: the healthiest country by 2020 – the report of the national preventative health taskforce*. Canberra: Commonwealth of Australia.

Coveney, J. and O'Dwyer, L.A., 2009. Effects of mobility and location on food access. *Health and Place*, 15 (1), 45–55.

Crotty, P.A., Rutishauser, I.H., and Cahill, M., 1992. Food in low-income families. *Australian Journal of Public Health*, 16 (2), 168–174.

Department for International Development, 1999. *Sustainable livelihood guidance sheets*. London: Department forInternational Development.

Donkin, A.J., *et al.*, 2000. Mapping access to food in a deprived area: the development of price and availability indices. *Public Health Nutrition*, 3 (1), 31–38.

Dowler, E., 1997. Budgeting for food on a low income in the UK: the case of lone-parent families. *Food Policy*, 22 (5), 405–417.

Drewnowski, A. and Eichelsdoerfer, P., 2009. Can low-income americans afford a healthy diet? *Nutrition Today*, 44 (6), 246–249.

Drewnowski, A. and Specter, S.E., 2004. Poverty and obesity: the role of energy density and energy costs. *American Journal of Clinical Nutrition*, 79 (1), 6–16.

Ellaway, A. and Macintyre, S., 2000. Shopping for food in socially contrasting localities. *British Food Journal*, 102, 52–59.

Foley, W., *et al.*, 2010. An ecological analysis of factors associated with food insecurity in South Australia. *Public Health Nutrition*, 13 (2), 215–221.

Gallegos, D., Ellies, P., and Wright, J., 2008. Still there's no food! Food insecurity in a refugee population in Perth, Western Australia. *Nutrition and Dietetics*, 65 (1), 78–83.

Gatrell, A.C., Popay, J., and Thomas, C., 2004. Mapping the determinants of health inequalities in social space: can Bourdieu help us? *Health Place*, 10 (3), 245–257.

Glanville, N. and McIntyre, L., 2006. Diet quality of atlantic families headed by single mothers. *Canadian Journal of Dietetic Practice and Research*, 67 (1), 28–35.

Gucciardi, E., Celasun, N., and Stewart, D.E., 2004. Single-mother families in Canada. *Canadian Journal of Public Health*, 95 (1), 70–73.

Harrison, M.S., *et al.*, 2007. The increasing cost of the basic foods required to promote health in Queensland. *Medical Journal of Australia*, 186 (1), 9–14.

Kirkpatrick, S.I. and Tarasuk, V., 2007. Adequacy of food spending is related to housing expenditures among lower-income Canadian households. *Public Health Nutrition*, 10 (12), 1464–1473.

Kirkpatrick, S.I. and Tarasuk, V., 2008. Food insecurity is associated with nutrient inadequacies among Canadian adults and adolescents. *Journal of Nutrition*, 138 (3), 604–612.

Lunnay, B., Ward, P., and Borlagdan, J., in press. The practise and practice of Bourdieu: the application of social theory to youth alcohol research. *International Journal of Drug Policy*, doi:10.1016/j.drugpo.2011.07.013.

Marks, G.C., *et al.*, 2001. *Key food and nutrition data for Australia 1990-1999*. Canberra: Commonwealth of Australia.

Martin, K.S. and Ferris, A.M., 2007. Food insecurity and gender are risk factors for obesity. *Journal of Nutrition Education and Behavior*, 39 (1), 31–36.

McIntyre, L., 2003. Food security: more than a determinant of health. *Policy Options*, 24 (3), 46–51.

McIntyre, L., *et al.*, 2002. Food insecurity of low-income lone mothers and their children in Atlantic Canada. *Canadian Journal of Public Health*, 93 (6), 411–415.

McIntyre, L., *et al.*, 2003a. Do low-income lone mothers compromise their nutrition to feed their children? *CMAJ*, 168 (6), 686–691.

McIntyre, L., Officer, S., and Robinson, L.M., 2003b. Feeling poor: the felt experience low-income lone mothers. *Affilia*, 18 (3), 316–331.

McLaughlin, C., Tarasuk, V., and Kreiger, N., 2003. An examination of at-home food preparation activity among low-income, food-insecure women. *Journal of the American Dietetic Association*, 103 (11), 1506–1512.

National Preventative Health Taskforce, 2009. *Australia: the healthiest country by 2020*. Canberra: Commonwealth of Australia.

Page, M.E. and Stevens, A.H., 2004. The economic consequences of absent parents. *Journal of Human Resources*, 39 (1), 80–107.

Polit, D.F., London, A.S., and Martinez, J.M., 2000. *Food security and hunger in poor, mother-headed families in four U.S. cities. The project on devolution and urban change working paper*. New York, NY: Manpower Demonstration Research Corporation.

Ritchie, J. and Spencer, L., 1994. Qualitative data analysis for applied policy research. *In*: A. Bryman and R. Burgess, eds. *Analyzing qualitative data*. London: Sage, 173–194.

Rychetnik, L., *et al.*, 2003. *Food security options paper: A planning framework and menu of options for policy and practice interventions*. Sydney: NSW Centre for Public Health Nutrition.

Sayer, A., 2005. *The moral significance of class*. Cambridge, MA: Cambridge University Press.

Seligman, H.K., *et al.*, 2007. Food insecurity is associated with diabetes mellitus: results from the national health examination and nutrition examination survey (NHANES) 1999–2002. *Journal of General Internal Medicine*, 22 (7), 1018–1023.

Sen, A., 1999. *Development as freedom*. New York: Knopf.

Serrat, O., 2010. *The livelihoods framework* [online]. Tokyo, Asian Development Bank. Available from: http://www.adb.org/Projects/Tonle_Sap/presentations.asp [Accessed 13 January 2011].

Shannon, C., 2002. Acculturation: Aboriginal and Torres Strait Islander nutrition. *Asia Paciific Journal of Clinical Nutrition*, 11 (Suppl 3), S576–S578.

Shilling, C., 1993. *The body and social theory*. London: Sage.

Silverman, D., 2001. *Interpreting qualitative data: Methods for analysing talk, text and interaction*. 2nd ed. London: Sage.

Stevens, C.A., 2010. Exploring food insecurity among young mothers (15–24 years). *Journal for Specialists in Pediatric Nursing*, 15 (2), 163–171.

Tarasuk, V., 2001. A critical examination of community-based responses to household food insecurity in Canada. *Health Education and Behavior*, 28 (4), 487–499.

Tarasuk, V. and Vogt, J., 2009. Household food insecurity in Ontario. *Canadian Journal of Public Health*, 100 (3), 184–188.

Townsend, M.S., *et al.*, 2001. Food insecurity is positively related to overweight in women. *Journal of Nutrition*, 131 (6), 1738–1745.

Turrell, G. and Kavanagh, A.M., 2006. Socio-economic pathways to diet: modelling the association between socio-economic position and food purchasing behaviour. *Public Health Nutrition*, 9 (3), 375–383.

Vozoris, N.T. and Tarasuk, V.S., 2003. Household food insufficiency is associated with poorer health. *Journal of Nutrition*, 133 (1), 120–126.

Wardle, J. and Baranovic, M., 2009. Is lack of retail competition in the grocery sector a public health issue? *Australian and New Zealand Journal of Public Health*, 33 (5), 477–481.

Women and Economic Development Consortium, 2001. *Women in transition out of poverty*. Toronto: Women and Economic Development Consortium.

Wong, K.C., *et al.*, 2011. Availability, affordability and quality of a healthy food basket in Adelaide, South Australia. *Nutrition and Dietetics*, 68 (1), 8–14.

Doing 'healthier' food in everyday life? A qualitative study of how Pakistani Danes handle nutritional communication

Bente Halkier and Iben Jensen

Department of Communication, Business and Information Technologies,
Roskilde University, Roskilde, Denmark

Denmark has a strong tradition of public health communication, but the majority of these initiatives draw upon the deficit model where the so called target groups are seen as passive recipients that lack resources to change their lifestyle. The article contributes to the critique of the deficit model in public health communication by the way of two steps. First, by arguing in favour of using a contextual theoretical perspective, that includes multiple social conditions and dynamics, a combination of practice theory and intersectionality. Second, by presenting an ideal-typology of ways of doing 'healthier' food among Pakistani Danes, based on a qualitative empirical study of food habits, everyday life and dealings with nutritional communication.

Introduction

Denmark has a strong tradition of public health promotion in the food consumption area via information campaigns and dietary advice (Vallgårda 2001). But a majority of the Danish dietary advice and communication campaigns about a healthy diet usually do not consider how food is embedded in the multiple social relations and conditions of everyday life. Typically, dietary advice and communication campaigns also do not take into account what the resources of the particular target group are. Or rather, it is assumed that the target group lacks resources to carry out the changes of habits that are being communicated.

These two characteristics of the bulk of communication campaigns about healthier food habits are based on the traditional sender–receiver model in communication (McQuail 1998, Jensen 2002, Craig 2007). From this perspective, users of informational advice and communication campaigns are seen as passive receivers of knowledge, values, and guidelines. One specific version of the traditional sender–receiver framework is called 'the deficit model'. It highlights the lack of resources among receivers in addition to the passive character of receiving (Hansen et al. 2003, Eden 2009). In other words, members of the specific target group are typically seen as lacking correct knowledge or lacking the 'right' attitudes in order to change their behaviour in the communicated direction. Ethnic minorities are characterised as having even fewer resources due to loss of social relations, cultural points of reference, mother tongue in communication, social status, national membership, community membership, meaning of life, and happiness (Mygind 2006). In this way the existing public intercultural health communication can be described as a double-deficit approach (Jensen and Halkier 2011).

This type of public communication has also been criticised on the basis of empirical research in the field of public health for being unrealistic in relation to achieving healthier everyday practices, as well as being disrespectful and potentially disempowering in relation to citizens (Holm 2003, Green 2008, Hankivsky and Christoffersen 2008, Carlisle and Cropper 2009, Sulkunen 2009, Lindsay 2010). The critics of the deficit model argue that food practices are embedded in the social and practical complexities of everyday life, and what healthier eating might consist in and how to do it is constructed differently in different social relations, situations, and fields of activity. In order to grasp the complexities of people's dealings with health recommendations in everyday life, a contextual perspective that includes multiple social conditions and dynamics is needed (Hankivsky and Christoffersen 2008, pp. 275–276).

In this article, we contribute to the critique of the deficit model in public health communication in two ways. We build upon a contextual theoretical perspective, and we present an empirical typology of ways of handling official nutritional guidelines among Pakistani Danes. The empirical typology shows that there are variations and multiplexity in mundane practical and normative[1] regulation of 'healthier'[2] food practicing, even within a relatively narrowly defined target group of citizens, in this case a minority ethnic group of Danes. The article is structured as follows: first, we position the argumentation of the article in relation to the Danish context of food and health and in relation to the international literature in the field. Second, we clarify our theoretical basis in practice theory and the methodological design of the empirical study. Third, the typology of ways of handling official nutritional guidelines is presented.

Rationalised and individualised 'healthier' food

The Danish tradition of public food information has become increasingly nutritionalised and individualised (Holm 2003). The most important public institution in this respect is the Agency of Consumer Affairs, which since 1936 has informed the general Danish population about what is considered proper nutrition. A diachronic text analysis of information campaign material from the Agency of Consumer Affairs to households from 1936 to 1985 shows that proper nutrition became increasingly and exclusively discursively framed as prevention of specific modern lifestyle and food-related diseases, such as obesity. As a part of this development, proper food practices were constructed as being based upon scientific nutritional knowledge and rational planning rather than other everyday consider-ations such as satiety, economic resources, taste preferences, and cooking skills. Also, communication about food practices became targeted to individuals as the ones to be nutritionally regulated, rather than families and communities (Christensen 1998).

In a more recent comparative European study, the tendency to individualise the responsibility for a nutritionally healthier diet in Denmark was also reflected. An analysis of the understanding of the food consumer among a broad variety of representatives of societal actors in the food sector – producers, manufacturers, retailers, public authorities, scientists, media, and consumer organisations – in four European countries[3] showed that in relation to nutrition and health, all types of actors in Denmark ascribed the main responsibility to individual consumers themselves (Halkier et al. 2007, p. 389). Also, in comparison with other Scandinavian countries, Danish preventive lifestyle policies are individualised (Vallgårda 2007).

The latest big initiative in public health in Denmark was the report launched by the Danish Commission for Prevention on diet, smoking, alcohol and exercise (Forebyggelseskommissionen 2009). The recommendations for public health initiatives in the report fall in two types in all four areas: individually targeted regulations such as taxes and prohibitions, and regulations targeted towards communities and institutions such as school lunches. In the area of dietary recommendations, there are nearly twice as many individually targeted initiatives as there are initiatives targeted towards communities and institutions.

New target groups, such as ethnic minority Danes, become included in this kind of individualised official public health initiatives on food. Pakistani Danes become particularly targeted, because they have a comparatively high risk of getting Type 2 diabetes and coronary heart disease, which is characteristic of this social group also in other national contexts (Bush et al. 1998, Mellin-Olsen and Wandel 2005, Ristovski-Slijepcevic et al. 2008). But in communication to and with ethnic minority Danes about healthier diets, social and cultural conditions and resources are seldom taken into account (Jensen and Halkier 2011).[4] In the following quote from our empirical case study – which we will present later – two Pakistani Danish women discuss the type of dietary advice people in their social networks who are diagnosed with Type 2 diabetes have experienced:

> Rushy[5]: The problem is when there is an interpreter, right, people who get this kind of diabetes, they get sent to Gentofte or out to Klampenborg somewhere there's a centre, right, and then this sort of dietician turns up and tells you about rye bread and dairy products, mayonnaise and tartare sauce and such things.
> Ishiita: We can't really use that for anything.

The reported experience is that dieticians give advice that is based on majority Danish food habits, which include rye bread, dairy products and mayonnaise. The women's conclusion is quite clear: they cannot really use that sort of advice. Studies from other national contexts with Pakistani minority citizens show similar patterns: that even in direct dietary communication between, for example, health workers and patients with minority ethnic background, the minority cultural food traditions are not acknowledged (Fagerli et al. 2005, p. 299).

A number of studies in the current international literature on food and health view food provisioning, cooking, and eating as practical activities that are socially and symbolically organised and entangled in the conditions, resources, relations, and negotiations of everyday life (e.g. Coveney 2000, Jabs and Devine 2006, Bava et al. 2008, Ristovski-Slijepcevic et al. 2008, Delormier et al. 2009). That is the perspective on which this article is based. This perspective is quite different from other strands in the current literature that are based on cognitivist approaches, such as the theory of planned behaviour (e.g. Aikman et al. 2006, Fishbein and

Capella 2006, Blanchard *et al.* 2009). In cognitivist studies, changes of food habits in healthier directions are assumed to result from obtaining more information, parallel to the assumptions in the 'deficit model'.

In the next two sections, the specific theoretical framework and the methodological design in our empirical case study are briefly presented.

Practice theory and intersectionality

A practice theoretical perspective is a particular reading of an assembly of theoretical elements from, among others, early Pierre Bourdieu (1990), Judith Butler (1990), early Anthony Giddens (1984), and late Michel Foucault (1978). The shared assumptions among these theoreticians about how social action is carried out and carried through are central in practice theory. Recent conceptual systematisation (Reckwitz 2002, Schatzki 2002, Warde 2005) turns the elements into a distinct analytical approach to the performativity of social life. A much-quoted definition of the concept of practice is the following:

> A practice … is a routinised type of behaviour which consists of several elements, interconnected to one other: forms of bodily activities, forms of mental activities, things and their use, a background knowledge in the form of understanding, know-how, states of emotion and motivational knowledge. A practice – a way of cooking, of consuming, of working, of investigating, of taking care of oneself or of other etc. – forms so to speak a 'block' whose existence necessarily depends on the existence and specific interconnectedness of these elements, and which cannot be reduced to any one of these single elements (Reckwitz 2002, pp. 249–250).

In the sociology of consumption, analytical 'translations' of the practice theoretical approach have been produced in order to make the concepts more operative in relation to empirical research in, for example, food practices. Alan Warde (2005, p. 14) clarifies the concept of practice as constituting a nexus of practical activity and its representations (doings and sayings), which become coordinated by understandings, procedures, and engagements. Understandings are the practical interpretations of what and how to do; knowledge and know-how in a broad sense. Procedures are instructions, principles, and rules of how to do. Engagements are emotional and normative orientations related to what and how to do. Each of the three elements that coordinate practices – understandings, procedures and engagements – comprises both tacit as well as discursive processes, and they cover bodily as well as mental processes. The characteristics of a particular practice, such as eating or cooking, are the qualities of the routinely repeated activities and their coordinating elements – understandings, procedures and engagements – rather than qualities of the individual food practitioner (Warde 2005, pp. 133–135).

Each individual participates in many different intersecting practices in his or her everyday contexts, whereby the different normative expectations connected to the performing of each practice create negotiations among practitioners about how to behave properly. The practice theoretical approach enables us to analyse the unfolding of practical morality in everyday practices among food practitioners as they enact and negotiate acceptable and expectable food conduct. To eat 'healthier food' or to cook 'a good meal' are not essential categories but rather contextual and often negotiated accomplishments among practitioners in intersections between food practices and many other practices; for example, job practices, mothering practices and socialising practices. Such processes of continuous practical and discursive accomplishments of conduct are what we call 'doing healthier food'. This perspective is inspired by the intersectionality approaches (e.g. Collins 2000, Fenstermaker and West 2002, Salih and Butler 2004) that share some of the assumptions of practice theory, such as the processual performative character of social life and the multi-relational character of the conditions of social life. For example, Hankivsky and Christoffersen (2008) argue on the basis of an intersectionality approach that health determinants and inequalities in health relate to complicated and dynamic intersections of aspects such as class, gender and ethnicity in everyday life conditions and practices. In our empirical case study with Pakistani Danes, 'doing healthier food' is continuously done, re-done, adapted, negotiated, and experimented within intersections of different practices, relations and conditions such as mothering practices and socialising practices.

Research design

The empirical research drawn upon in this article is a qualitative in-depth study of the food habits of ethnic Pakistani Danes and how 'doing healthy food' is handled among them. The overall selective sampling strategy was one of maximum variation regarding the following criteria: age (15–65); education (with and without high school degree); gender; whether participants were born in Denmark or Pakistan; whether a person in the family had been diagnosed with diabetes 2; and whether participants worked in the health sector. A total of 19 Pakistani Danes participated in individual interviews, family interviews or group interviews.

The qualitative data in this study were produced by several methods. One part of the data was produced through individual in-depth interviews (Spradley 1979, Holstein and Gubrium 2003) with the main cooking practitioner in the family interviewed about provisioning, cooking and eating in their everyday life, in relation to other people in their network, and in relation to constructions of healthy food. Another part of the data was produced by auto-photography (Heisley and Levy 1991) of food and drinks consumed during weekdays and the weekend. The photos were used as data in themselves and as input in family interviews and group interviews (Frey and Fontana 1993). During all of these interviews, which were held in the home of the family, participant observation (Hammersley and Atkinson 1995) was also used.

The analysis of the data material was done by using ordinary qualitative coding and categorising (Coffey and Atkinson 1996); visual data analysis techniques (Hurdley 2007) and positioning analysis (Harré and Langenhove 1998), combined with the more operative concepts from practice theory. The categories and types based on the data material were also constructed in relation to intersectionality analysis, as all practices are intersected by more general social categories such as ethnicity, age and gender (Collins 2000). Furthermore, food practices are intersected by more specific social categories such as 'good cooking' and 'unhealthy food'. Food practices are also intersected with other everyday life practices such as job practices, socialising practices and family practices .The ideal-types presented in the following section were constructed on the basis of all the data, but in this article we mainly draw on the interview material in the presentation of the types.

Ways of doing 'healthier' food

In this section, an ideal typology of variations of doing healthier food is presented. We suggest on the basis of our empirical analysis that at least four different ideal-typical ways of doing healthier food can be constructed. The four ideal-types are: I: *Engaging proactively in healthier food;* II: *Fitting in healthier food;* III: *Doing healthier food ambivalently; and* IV: *Ignoring healthier food as social practicality.*

The ideal-types are related to practices, and not to specific individuals. Each of the types (ways of doing healthier food) in the ideal typology is performed by multiple participants. Likewise, every participant conducts food practices as shifting or gliding between several ways of doing healthier food in different contexts or relations, and each participant performs multiple food practices in one context. In methodological terms, the typology is not based on methodological individualism. This means that each of the types in the typology represents enactments from several participants, and the enactments of each individual participant may align with different ways of doing healthier food. In other words, the ideal typology represents inferences made about the performances of social categories of food practicing – and not about individual food practitioners.

Each ideal-type is presented in accordance with the practice theoretical perspective. First, activities done in a practice, 'doings and sayings', are described. Second, 'understandings', 'procedures', and 'engagement' for doing healthy food in relation to the different ideal-types are presented. Third, examples of multiplicity and contradiction in doing healthier food are highlighted.

Ideal-type I: Engaging proactively in healthier food

In this ideal-type, the activities (doing and sayings) consist in enactments of how what is constructed as healthier food is made and talked about. There are references to all the main elements of public Danish dietary advice: more vegetables and fruit, more fish, more whole grain products, less sugar and less animal fat (Andersson and Bryngelsson 2007, pp. 36–38). The 'understandings' of healthiness of cooking and eating are taken for granted, normatively.

Examples of cooking 'procedures' constructed as healthier are to make chicken, fish and kebab in the oven instead of in a pot or pan in order to use less oil; to steam vegetables instead of roasting them for a long time in a curry in order to maintain more vitamins; and to make 'biriani' instead of 'pilao'[6] in order to use less oil. In this example, one of the food practitioners describes how she makes her chicken, marinated in yogurt and spices:

> But it's usually that chicken in the oven. [. . .]Because the only thing is just to peel off the skin of the chicken. Some people make it with the skin, but as I've told you, I prefer not to because of all that fat. So, you know, off with the skin, and it also becomes better marinated. It gives more taste of the spices instead of the skin just getting it. (Sada, female nurse).

This means that the procedures of cooking activities have been changed in order to make what is constructed as healthier food in modern nutritional terms. This is parallel to a discourse called 'the mainstream healthy eating discourse' analysed among Punjabis in a Canadian study (Ristovski-Slijepcevic *et al.* 2008, pp. 72–73). However, using the oven is at the same time constructed as a way of saving and flexing time (Southerton 2006) spent on cooking. So cooking 'healthier' also accomplishes cooking more conveniently, which again provides time for other practices such as helping children with homework. Such multiplicity in practicing healthier food and intersectings with other social categories and practices can be analysed across the four different ideal-types.

Eating activities and procedures have been changed too. Food practitioners explain, for example, that they have cut down on how often they eat the traditional Pakistani breakfast meal parathas. This is a flat bread or thick pancake made by puff-paste, roasted in butter on a pan and buttered once again before eating. Typically, food practitioners eat it only on weekends, instead of every morning, and to avoid this, food is constructed as reflecting and taking care of your body:

> The whole family eats it, emh I think parathas are a bit heavy, I like the dry ones better, gradually a lot of people ... you know, those who are conscious about their bodies, they probably don't eat them so often. They love them, but they don't eat them so often. (Rushy, female academic).

Pakistani Danish guest food is understood as tasteful but also unhealthy due to the high contents of fat and sugar. Thus, the food practitioners find ways of handling these situations. Here is an exchange about such procedures from one of the family interviews where the two women (Sada, female nurse, and her sister-in-law Maria, female pedagogue) have just discussed scraping off oil from dishes:

> Interviewer: Is it allowed to take it off when you are at parties and so?
> Sada: We try.
> Maria: With quick movements! [showing with her hands]
> Sada: But you cannot avoid it. I can feel that it's probably one of the cheap kinds of fat that is usually being used in that sort of food.

In this ideal-type, the 'engagement' in healthier food is considerable. New knowledge about what is healthy and what is not healthy is questioned, discussed and actively pursued in magazines, books, from television shows and the Internet, and from other people in the social network. Communication and negotiation about food in a health context and serving of healthier dishes is being initiated both with members of the 'in-group' – mothers, daughters, sisters and sisters-in-law – but also with members of the larger social network.

Ideal-type II: Fitting in healthier food

This way of doing healthier food can be distinguished from the first type by the focus among practitioners on what is practically do-able. The activities in this ideal-type and the way of dealing with public food advice revolve around the practicalities of tacitly adjusting some of the 'procedures' in daily food practices to become healthier. Knowledge about healthier food is gained from books, television, Internet, cooking programmes, and the children's schools. 'Understandings' of nutrition and healthy food are taken for granted as something that is already a part of the activities of food practitioners. One of the husbands from a family interview puts it like this:

> Actually, we know already really well what is healthy and what is not healthy ... And we also try to make that, so actually we don't have to seek any advice ... But we do what we can. (Ahmed, male taxi driver).

The 'engagement' in doing healthy food is in this ideal-type expressed in the way food practitioners tacitly adapt some of their cooking and eating 'procedures', e.g. to bake chapattis with wholemeal flour. There is not as much discussion and communication going on as in the first ideal-type, but it seems on the other hand to be socially legitimate to talk about it with people in the intimate circles of the social network. One of the food practitioners explains after having been asked if she serves her less oily masalas for guests:

> Then we just tell them that this is what we have made and that here in our home we don't use very much oil. And that's how it is. (Shabana, female schoolteacher).

However, fitting in healthier food can also be part of a struggle of the power over family meals, enacted on the basis of reproduction of gender relations (Fenstermaker and West 2002). Solejma (female office clerk) explains that she is frustrated about her sister-in-law making dishes with lots of fat and sugar to her brother who is diagnosed with diabetes 2:

> You know, I tried (ehm) to explain to her from these leaflets my brother has from the organisation about (ehm) how he has to relate to food and what he must eat and what he should not (ehm), and tried to explain it to her. This is just where it goes wrong, that she doesn't understand what is written in these leaflets and catalogues that my brother has got.

Trying to fit in healthier food for Solejma, who cooks low-fat food to her brother, is intersected with gender relations, family positionings and negotiations on proper Pakistani food.

Ideal-type III: Doing healthier food ambivalently

Contradictions characterise this way of doing healthier food. 'Understandings' of healthier food are in accordance with public Danish dietary advice, just like in the first two ideal-types; some of the same 'procedures' are practiced; and there is also 'engagement' in cooking and eating healthier dishes and meals. But other types of engagements in food practices are also important, so what is constructed as healthier food activities and procedures are incorporated in food practices when they do not conflict too much with the other types of engagement in food practices. One such type of engagement is the managing of family time around the production and consumption of meals. This ambivalence was described in one of the family interviews:

> Aysha: We don't eat so much take-away.
> Hussein: Because we hate that junk food.
> Aysha: We make it, even though we hardly have any time to cook when we come home. He's just arrived too.

The exchange shows the potential ambivalence between managing family time and cooking what is constructed as proper food and healthier meals. This potential ambivalence in doing healthier food was also performed another day when we unexpectedly visited Aysha's family to deliver a camera. When we arrived they were all enjoying eating take-away pizza for dinner, showing us how to 'spice it up', while simultaneously insistently explaining that this kind of dinner happened very rarely. A further interpretation of the examples is that they seem to reflect the dilemmas of providing proper food related to intersectings of gender, ethnicity and health. Take-away pizza can be necessary because of the gendered division of food labour in the family and Aysha's full-time job. Take-away pizza is also seen as unhealthy food to be avoided, because it is not homemade, but at the same time, such pizza can be made into more proper food by adding Pakistani spices.

Ideal-type IV: Ignoring healthier food as social practicality

Here, there is little normative 'engagement' in healthier food. Rather, the engagements in food practices revolve around the pleasures of food, around 'understandings' of appropriate Pakistani food, and around prioritising the practising of food as care and upholding family relations. Food practitioners know and reproduce elements of public Danish dietary advice such as the food pyramid.[7] But these understandings are not necessarily put into practical 'procedures' in their everyday life, since the other engagements fit the social relations around cooking and eating better.

Engagement in cooking as family care is a typical example. To be able to cater for every family member's individual needs is a way of showing family love and reproducing the bonds within the family (Holm 2004, Moisio et al. 2004). Here the teenage daughter of Zabel, female kitchen worker, interprets her mother's caregiving understanding of cooking:

> You know, all of us are a bit spoiled, right. You know, a lot of times when my brother comes home from work, or maybe just suddenly at 11 o'clock in the evening, then he just feels like eating French fries or something like that, right. So sometimes he makes it himself, but he also says, mum, I need to have something now at eleven o'clock, and then she has to make it.

For Zabel it is more important to make the food that her son loves than to make a healthier dish. From the perspective of intersectionality, this example at the same time clearly shows how all social actions are intersected by gender, age and power (Collins 2000). Traditional gender is reconstructed in this example, as mother and son at the same time draw upon traditional gender relations.

Across ideal-types

As mentioned above, these ideal-types are related to practices and not to individuals. This means that to use the oven, avoid parathas, seek information on the Internet and serve fat free and sugar free cakes at parties do *not* mean that fish fingers and French fries are not served on an ordinary Tuesday, or that parathas are not enjoyed thoroughly on a Saturday morning. Across all the social differences among the participants in the research project, the pleasure of the taste of good food is never questioned. Food practitioners who enact engagement in healthier food and specific procedures for how to cook e.g. with less fat also enact how unpleasant and inappropriate healthier food can be. Here is an example where one of the food practitioners, Maria, Sada's sister-in-law, gives an account of her own sister's cooking, just after Sada has concluded that reduction of fat constitutes proper cooking:

> Sada: I never use fat.
> Maria: My sister, do you know what she does? She only uses two teaspoons [of oil], and then when the onions have coloured, she takes the oil out and throws it away. And then she finishes the dish, that's why her food tastes so bad. [. . .]
> Sada: That's not good. That definitely doesn't taste nice.

Maria: No, it doesn't taste good, but then she feels she has done a good deed, right... NOW we're eating healthy!

Thus, a gliding in the construction of the category of good cooking takes place: from food without fat to food with fat. Experiences from life trajectories of having learned how to cook and eat proper Pakistani food are negotiated in relation to ways of cooking nutritionally healthier food (Mellin-Olsen and Wandel 2005, p. 334).

Conclusion

In this article, we have contributed to the analytical critique of the deficit model in public health communication by drawing upon a theoretical perspective that includes multiple social dynamics and by presenting an empirical typology of different ways of doing healthier food among Pakistani Danes. In contrast to the implicit deficit model assumptions of much public health communication, ordinary food practitioners are shown to be knowledgeable and resourceful. Across the social differences among the participants in the study, the public dietary advices are well-known.

On the basis of the constructed ideal-types, our study suggests that public health communication should build upon the following ideas: First, users (food practitioners) are to be seen as knowing and resourceful – which is in contrast to the implicit deficit model assumption. Second, communication strategies towards ideal-types II and III need to be focusing upon practices that are easy to fit into a modern, busy, everyday life. Third, it might be possible to suggest new, time-consuming and at the same time healthier food practices – like making less unhealthy snacks from scratch – as use of time indicates caring in this ideal-type.

However, the food practitioners also strive to accomplish healthier food in intersections of many different practicalities, food engagements, expectations in network relations, and socio-cultural conditions. The variety of ways of doing healthier food, and the multiplicities and negotiations of the categories of 'good' food show that it is never the belonging to just one category that explains health-related patterns in everyday life. Even in this relatively narrowly defined target group, there is quite a lot of variation and complexity in the practical and social regulation of how to cook and eat healthier.

Acknowledgement

The research project 'Network communication and changes in food practices – a case-study of food habits and social network among ethnic Pakistani Danes in risk of diabetes 2' was financed by the National Danish Social Science Research Council (FSE), 2008 – 2010.

Notes

1. We use the term 'normative' instead of 'moral', because 'normative' is related to social norms. Social norms are more specific, practical, and flexible ways of regulating human conduct than moral values, which are often more general and abstract and tend to be treated as more rule-bound (Mortensen 1992).
2. Healthier' here is understood as the current official Danish nutritional advice (Andersson and Bryngelsson 2007, pp. 36–38).
3. Denmark, Italy, Norway and Portugal.
4. A notable exception in Denmark is the education programme in some of the local municipalities called 'Healthy in your own language', where representatives from different

ethnic minority groups get a short education in order to work as 'health ambassadors' in their own social networks afterwards, based on 'peer-to-peer' principles.

5. The participants in the case study have been given pseudonyms in order to preserve their anonymity.
6. In biriani, the roasted ingredients (vegetables, spices etc.) are mixed into the steamed rice just before being served, whereas in pilao, the rice is roasted together with the other ingredients, requiring more oil in order not to stick to the pot.
7. The food pyramid has staples in the bottom, vegetables and fruit in the middle, and meat, eggs and dairy products in the top. The advice is to eat most from the bottom and least from the top.

References

Aikman, S., Min, K.E., and Graham, D., 2006. Food attitudes, eating behavior, and the information underlying food attitudes. *Appetite*, 47, 111–114.

Andersson, A. and Bryngelsson, S., 2007. Towards a healthy diet: from nutrition recommendations to dietary advice. *Scandinavian Journal of Food and Nutrition*, 51, 31–40.

Bava, C.M., Jaeger, S.R., and Park, J., 2008. Constraints upon food provisioning practices in 'busy' women's lives: trade-offs which demand convenience. *Appetite*, 50, 486–498.

Blanchard, C.M., *et al.*, 2009. Do ethnicity and gender matter when using the theory of planned behavior to understand fruit and vegetable consumption? *Appetite*, 52, 15–20.

Bourdieu, P., 1990. *The logic of practice*. Cambridge: Polity Press.

Bush, H., *et al.*, 1998. Family hospitality and ethnic tradition among South Asian, Italian and General Population Women in the West of Scotland. *Sociology of Health and Illness*, 20, 351–380.

Butler, J., 1990. *Gender trouble. feminism and the subversion of identity*. New York: Routledge.

Carlisle, S. and Cropper, S., 2009. Investing in lay researchers for community-based health action research: implications for research, policy and practice. *Critical Public Health*, 19, 59–70.

Christensen, G., 1998. *Diskursiv Regulering af Ernæringspraksis* (Discursive regulation of dietary practice). Thesis (PhD). The Royal Veterinary and Agricultural University.

Coffey, A. and Atkinson, P., 1996. *Making sense of qualitative data*. London: Sage.

Collins, P.H., 2000. *Black feminist thought: knowledge, consciousness and the politics of empowerment*. New York: Routledge.

Coveney, J., 2000. *Food, morals and meaning. The pleasure and anxiety of eating*. London: Routledge.

Craig, R., 2007. Communication theory as a field. *In*: R.T. Craig and H.L. Muller, eds. *Theorizing communication: Readings across traditions*. London: Sage, 63–98.

Delormier, T., Frohlich, K.L., and Potvin, L., 2009. Food and eating as social practice – understanding eating patterns as social phenomena and implications for public health. *Sociology of Health and Illness*, 31, 215–228.

Eden, S., 2009. Food labels as boundary objects: how consumers make sense of organic and functional foods. *Public Understanding of Science*, 18, 1–16.

Fagerli, R.Å., Lien, M.E., and Wandel, M., 2005. Experience of dietary advice among Pakistani-born persons with type 2 diabetes in Oslo. *Appetite*, 45, 295–304.

Fenstermaker, S. and West, C., 2002. *Doing gender, doing difference. inequality, power and institutional change*. New York: Routledge.

Fishbein, M. and Capella, J.N., 2006. The role of theory in developing effective health communications. *Journal of Communication*, 56, 1–17.

Forebyggelseskommisionen, 2009. *Vi kan Leve Længere og Sundere* [We can live longer and healthier]. Copenhagen.

Foucault, M., 1978. *The history of sexuality*. Vol. 1, Harmondsworth: Penguin.

Frey, J.H. and Fontana, A., 1993. The group interview in social research. *In*: D.L. Morgan, ed. *Successful focus groups*. London: Sage, 20–34.

Giddens, A., 1984. *The constitution of society*. Cambridge: Polity Press.

Green, J., 2008. Health education – the case for rehabilitation. *Critical Public Health*, 18, 447–456.

Halkier, B., *et al.*, 2007. Trusting, complex, quality conscious or unprotected? Constructing the food consumer in different European national contexts. *Journal of Consumer Culture*, 7, 295–318.

Hammersley, M. and Atkinson, P., 1995. *Ethnography. Principles in practice*. London: Routledge.

Hankivsky, O. and Christoffersen, A., 2008. Intersectionality and the determinants of health: a Canadian perspective. *Critical Public Health*, 18, 271–283.

Hansen, J., *et al.*, 2003. Beyond the knowledge deficit: recent research into lay and expert attitudes to food risks. *Appetite*, 41, 111–121.

Harré, R. and Langenhove, L., 1998. *Positioning theory*. Oxford: Blackwell.

Heisley, D.D. and Levy, S.J., 1991. Autodriving: photoelicitation technique. *Journal of Consumer Research*, 18 (3), 257–272.

Holm, L., 2003. Blaming the consumer: on the free choice of consumers and the decline in food quality in Denmark. *Critical Public Health*, 13, 139–154.

Holm, L., 2004. Måltidet som Socialt Fællesskab [The meal as community]. *In*: L. Holm, ed. *Mad, Mennesker og Måltider – Samfundsvidenskabelige Perspektiver [Food, people and meals – social scientific perspectives]*. København: Munksgaard.

Holstein, J.A. and Gubrium, J.F., 2003. Active interviewing. *In*: J.F. Gubrium and J.A. Holstein, eds. *Postmodern interviewing*. London: Sage, 148–161.

Hurdley, R., 2007. Focal points: framing material culture and visual data. *Qualitative Research*, 7 (3), 355–374.

Jabs, J. and Devine, C.M., 2006. Time scarcity and food choices: an overview. *Appetite*, 47, 196–204.

Jensen, I. and Halkier, B., 2011. Rethinking intercultural network communication as a resource in public intercultural health communication. *Journal of Intercultural Communication*, 25, 1.

Jensen, K.B., 2002. *A handbook of media and communication research*. London: Routledge.

Lindsay, J., 2010. Healthy living guidelines and the disconnect with everyday life. *Critical Public Health*, 20, 475–487.

Mellin-Olsen, T. and Wandel, M., 2005. Changes in food habits among Pakistani immigrant women in Oslo, Norway. *Ethnicity and Health*, 10, 311–339.

McQuail, D., 1998. *Audience analysis*. London: Sage.

Moisio, R., Arnould, E.J., and Price, L.L., 2004. Between mothers and markets: Constructing family identity through homemade food. *Journal of Consumer Culture*, 4 (3), 361–384.

Mortensen, N., 1992. Future norms. *In*: P. Gundelach and K. Siune, eds. *From voters to participants*. Aarhus: Politica.

Mygind, A., *et al.*, 2006. *Etniske minoriteters opfattelse af sygdomsrisici – betydningen af etnicitet og migration* [Ethnic minorities' understanding of health risks – the influence of ethnicity and migration], København: *Sundhedsstyrelsen* [National Health Board].

Reckwitz, A., 2002. Toward a theory of social practices. A development in culturalist theorizing. *European Journal of Social Theory*, 5 (2), 243–263.

Ristovski-Sliepevic, S., Chapman, G.E., and Beagan, B.L., 2008. Engaging with healthy eating discourse(s): ways of knowing about food and health in three ethnocultural groups in Canada. *Appetite*, 50, 167–178.

Salih, S. and Butler, J., 2004. *The Judith Butler reader*. Oxford: Blackwell Publishing.

Schatzki, T.R., 2002. *The site of the social: a philosophical account of the constitution of social life and change*. Pennsylvania State University Press, University Park, PA.

Southerton, D., 2006. Analysing the temporal organization of daily life: social constraints, practices and their allocation. *Sociology*, 40, 435–54.

Spradley, J.P., 1979. *The ethnographic interview*. Fort Worth: Holt, Rinehart and Winston.

Sulkunen, P., 2009. *The Saturated society: governing risk and lifestyles in consumer culture*. London: Sage.

Vallgårda, S., 2001. Governing people's lives. Strategies for improving the health of the nations in England, Denmark, Norway and Sweden. *European Journal of Public Health*, 11, 386–392.

Vallgårda, S., 2007. Health inequalities: political problematizations in Denmark and Sweden. *Critical Public Health*, 17, 45–56.

Warde, A., 2005. Consumption and theories of practice. *Journal of Consumer Culture*, 5 (2), 131–153.

A focus group study of food safety practices in relation to listeriosis among the over-60s

Richard Milne

Department of Geography, University of Sheffield, Sheffield, UK

In recent years, policy attention has moved from the safety of food at the point of sale to focus on the roles and responsibilities of the consumer in managing food risks. Although the redefinition of consumer roles and responsibilities has taken place across the board, responsibilities for risk management and avoidance are not equally distributed, as some consumers are significantly more 'vulnerable' than others to food-borne illnesses. Nevertheless, vulnerability to food poisoning does not immediately equate with being 'at risk'. Orienting itself primarily to the example of listeriosis in the over-60s, this article draws on the early findings of current qualitative research into older people's attitudes to food and use of date labels to consider the relationship between vulnerability and food safety risk. It situates this study within a review of existing studies of food choice in later life to argue for its relevance to food safety policy. It suggests that this can best be developed by adopting an approach that draws on theories of social practice.

Introduction

Eating involves potential exposure to an astonishing range of food-borne illnesses, from *Campylobacter* to *Salmonella*, *Escherichia coli*, *Norovirus* and vCJD. Each has a distinct epidemiology that makes it difficult to identify universal risk factors or relevant consumer practices. Moreover, not all people are equally susceptible to serious infection, with the elderly, pregnant and immuno-compromised, especially vulnerable to certain pathogens (Advisory Committee on the Microbiological Safety of Food; ACMSF 2009). Consequently, this article focuses on the production of consumer food safety risk in relation to one specific illness, listeriosis, among one particular group, the over-60s. It moves away from the problematisation of consumer behaviour as the 'weakest link in the food chain' (Terpstra *et al.* 2005, Brennan *et al.* 2007) to develop an understanding of the socially, historically and spatially embedded nature of food safety practices.

Caused by the bacterium *Listeria monocytogenes*, listeriosis is associated with particular foods and how they are used, including ready-to-eat foods with an extended, refrigerated shelf-life, such as prepared sandwiches, bagged salads, cut

fruit, hummus, smoked fish, pâté and soft cheese. *Listeria monocytogenes* populations in these foods are controlled during production and retail storage by the
maintenance of a 'cold chain' from manufacture to sale. Beyond this point, risks
emerge or are controlled through consumer food shopping and storage activities.
The 'correct' duration and conditions of storage are communicated in the form of the
'use-by' date and directions to 'store between 0°C and 5°C'.

Listeriosis is most common in the pregnant and new-born, the elderly and those
whose immune system has been compromised. Between 1990 and 2007, 2152 cases of
listeriosis were reported in the UK. However, between the late 1990s and 2007, rates
of listeriosis in the UK doubled, with the increase taking place almost exclusively in
the over-60s. This increase is paralleled by similar rises across Europe (Goulet *et al.*
2008). It is of particular concern as the infection is fatal in around 30% of cases in
the over-60s. In 2009, the *ad hoc* group on vulnerable groups of ACMSF (2009)
considered a number of possible causes, concluding that the changing epidemiology
was more likely to be linked to social factors, including changes in consumption
behaviour or in food production. However, a review by the FSA's Social Science
Research Committee (SSRC 2009) suggests no dramatic social changes can be
identified from existing evidence.

Knowledge and practice

Policy-oriented discussion of food safety risks and of listeriosis in particular have
concentrated on the links between food safety knowledge and food storage
behaviours (e.g. Cates *et al.* 2006, ACMSF 2009, Hutton 2009, SSRC 2009,
Gillespie *et al.* 2010a, b). In 2009, the FSA's Food Safety Week campaign attempted
to reduce the incidence of listeriosis by making older people aware of the dangers of
out-of-date food and the importance of keeping fridge temperatures below 5°C
(Hutton 2009). The campaign involved a series of educational leaflets and TV
adverts aimed at convincing rational consumers to reform unsafe food safety
behaviours. However, there is little evidence that such education and awareness
campaigns have the desired effect (Milton and Mullan 2010).

An alternative approach, to both analysis and intervention, may be developed by
drawing on theories of social practice, recently applied to food in the fields of
shopping (Everts and Jackson 2009), cooking (Meah and Watson 2011), nutrition
(Halkier and Jensen 2011) and waste (Evans in press). Social practices are routinised
types of behaviours which consist of several interconnected elements: bodily and
mental activities; 'things' and their use; background understandings; know-how;
emotional states; and motivational knowledge (Reckwitz 2002, Warde 2005, Jackson
et al. 2006). For Shove and Pantzar (2010), these elements of practice can be reduced
to three groups: things (materials, technology); images (meanings, symbols) and
skills (competencies, procedures). Understood as practice, shopping for food is not
simply a question of acquiring provisions, nor is disposing of food only a matter of
safety. It involves the performance of complex and situated social roles and the
reproduction and maintenance of interrelations between these elements of practice.

Halkier and Jensen (2011) suggest that practice theory offers two analytical
affordances that are relevant to this study. The first positions both food practices
and food consumption activities within practices as 'flows of happenings and
processes of carrying out activities that are both productive and conditioned'

(Halkier and Jensen 2011, p. 105). This enables food safety to be approached as part of domestic activities of food provisioning, retention and disposal, collectively understood as making up food storage. These activities are carried out in the context of the wider institutional dynamics of food consumption. The second affordance is the recognition that the activities involved in practices, such as eating, shopping and cooking, must be continually re-done in order for a practice to persist. The maintenance of these practices thus represents an ongoing and precarious accomplishment, and food storage can be approached as a critical moment within the reproduction of social practices, rather than an isolated behaviour.

Seen through a social practice lens, the knowledge and know-how about food safety that are targeted by the FSA campaign represent only one part of the complex nexus of materials, competencies and images associated with everyday consumption. The application and relevance of knowledge is restrained by the configuration of the other components of practices. The following sections suggest that discussion of food safety in the over-60s in terms of food 'practices' offers the potential to develop new approaches and food safety interventions. Focussing on the heterogeneous components of 'food storage' practices, this article describes how food safety and listeriosis risk emerge within socially and geographically situated practices that exist in relation with other food-related routines, most importantly those of provisioning and disposal.

Food risk and the over-60s

Older people are more vulnerable to listeriosis (ACMSF 2009). However, while there has been significant interest in the food practices of older people in terms of nutrition and healthy eating (e.g. Herne 1995, McKie 1999, Lumbers and Raats 2006), little research has specifically considered food safety risks (although see Johnson *et al.* 1998). Food consumption in later life is subject to a range of changes (for reviews see Herne 1995, Lumbers and Raats 2006, Giles 2009). Many studies concentrate on the physical and mental changes associated with ageing, which remain among the most important influences on changes in food choice (Herne 1995). For example, sensory acuity decreases with age, making assessment on the basis of taste or smell potentially unreliable and the reading of labels difficult (Johnson *et al.* 1998). Declines in sight, hearing or dental health may result in problems with food preparation. In addition, conditions such as dementia may result in difficulties with food management, for example in forgetting how long a product has been in the fridge or to check dates (SSRC 2009).

McKie (1999, p. 535) suggests that older people 'may have to overcome a range of structural hurdles to continue to access the foods they have come to accept as part of their diet'. In the case of access to nutritive foods, research has described the existence of 'food deserts' (Wrigley 2002) areas within which access to cheap, fresh food is restricted, most commonly by the absence of large retailers. Although this term and its implications are contested (Cummins and McIntyre 2002), it highlights the potential consequences of changing food geographies for domestic consumption. In the past 50 years, the market share of the major supermarket retailers has risen from around 20% (1960) to well over 80% in 2010 (Cabinet Office 2008). Large supermarkets are often located on the outskirts of towns, or have primarily been designed for access by car. This is not in itself problematic for food safety, but becomes a potential problem in terms of domestic food storage when combined with restrictions on transport and mobility. Food shopping in many Western economies revolves around the use of cars. Access to and use of cars decreases dramatically with age, and is a major indicator of social exclusion among older people (Barnes *et al.* 2006). In 2006, 82% of women and 89% of men aged 60–69 in England had access to a car. However, among those aged 90 and over only 47% of women and 57% of men had access to a car, with only a small proportion driving them regularly (Barnes *et al.* 2006). Those without access to cars may be excluded and able to shop only infrequently (Herne 1995, Coveney and O'Dwyer 2009, Dean *et al.* 2009) or limited to more accessible shops within a smaller local area (Caraher *et al.* 1998, Turrini *et al.* 2010). This leads to decreased satisfaction with food shopping facilities (Bromley and Thomas 1993) and potentially the consumption of a narrower range of food (Banister and Bowling 2004, although see Wilson *et al.* 2004). Older people become increasingly dependent on informal networks in which others provide transport or shopping (Turrini *et al.* 2010). Moreover, the form of these alternatives affects store choice – older people are not necessarily able to access their preferred store. Indeed, it is only when transport is provided by family members rather than home-helps or neighbours that it is likely that people will purchase food from distant supermarkets rather than the same nearby 'convenience' stores (Lumbers and Raats 2006).

The potential relevance of this study to discussions of food safety is reflected by the findings of UK Health Protection Agency (HPA) work on listeriosis. For example, Gillespie *et al.* (2010b) draw on tracker data from market research agency TNS to examine the shopping patterns of listeriosis cases. They suggest that cases are more likely than the general population to purchase food at local 'convenience' stores (Gillespie *et al.* 2010b). Bringing this study together with the existing social science literature on older people's consumption patterns and new qualitative research enables this finding to be examined in more detail. This article suggests that the consequences of changing food practices are relevant for thinking about food safety as they are for nutrition, and that the separation of the two, now replicated in UK food policy, obscures insights into the factors that contribute to both.

Researching the food practices of older people

The research reported here involved six focus groups with older people recruited through existing social networks as part of a qualitative research project exploring how date labels and other forms of food safety information and behaviours are positioned within situated food safety practices. A focus group approach offers a number of advantages for this type of research, enabling participants to generate their own questions, frames and concepts and pursue their own priorities according to their own terms of reference (Kitzinger and Barbour 1999). Moreover, the focus group setting enables older people to participate who may have declined to take part in a one-to-one interview or ethnographic setting (cf. Jackson and Holbrook 1995). Contacting participants through existing social networks offers further advantages, both in encouraging participation and offering the potential for more 'naturalistic' discussions (Jackson and Holbrook 1995, Kitzinger 1995, Green *et al.* 2005).

Groups were conducted in Sheffield and Norfolk and were recruited through visits or in one case through contact with a trusted 'gatekeeper' who facilitated access to an existing group of which they were a member. The balance of groups in Sheffield and Norfolk allowed groups to be recruited in areas with differing socio-economic profiles and accounted for potential differences between urban and rural perspectives on food, although no significant differences emerged in the group discussions. The ages of participants ranged from 60 to 90.[1] The constituency and profile of the groups are summarised in Table 1.

The groups were provided with information on the study and were paid an incentive of £10 for their participation. Each group meeting lasted 90 minutes and followed a semi-structured protocol which explored attitudes and routines related to food in general and participants' use of food labelling. This protocol allowed participants to concentrate on their own concerns, or lack of, about food, including but not limited to safety. This approach reflected the finding of previous studies (e.g. Green *et al.* 2005) that safety, although important to people, is not a primary concern or focus of food-related attitudes. The focus groups were transcribed and analysed using NVivo. Common themes were identified in the data and used to develop a common coding framework across the group discussions. This provides the framework for the discussion in the following sections, which consider how the focus group data illustrate arguments about the geographically and socially situated nature of food practices of the over-60s. In particular, they explore the relations between the elements food storage practices as they emerge in focus group discussions. In doing so, they explore and extend the conclusion of Johnson *et al.* (1998) that food storage among elderly people does not minimise the risk of food poisoning.

Risky dispositions

A common popular narrative of older people's food practices often refers to the inculcation of thrift during the war and post-war years of austerity, and consequent reluctance to waste. Older people are described as more significantly concerned about food waste than other age groups (WRAP 2008) and consequently as lacking what has elsewhere been termed the 'disposition' (Maycroft 2009) for disposal. This is a stereotype that focus groups themselves repeat as they critique friends' and relatives' attitudes to food waste:

> D: *My granddaughter's dreadful. When she comes to stay she'll go through and she says 'Nan, that sell-by date', I say 'Put it back I'll eat that'*
> A: *My daughters-in-law are similar to that*
> D: *She's so dreadful with sell-by dates*

Table 1. Summary of focus groups.

Group	Location	N	Group description
A	Norfolk	8	Church group
B	N Sheffield	4	Resident's group
C	C Sheffield	8	Tenant's association
D	Norfolk	7	Allotment holders
E	NW Sheffield	4	Coffee morning
F	W Sheffield	3	Church group

*J: It's wasteful because we were brought up during the war when food was rationed so we
make the most of everything, I very rarely waste anything*
(Group E)

The experience of scarcity was important in shaping these participants' attitudes
to food storage and waste. In the vocabulary introduced earlier, these experiences
contribute to the formation of motivational states associated with food storage that
emphasise the avoidance of waste. However, as discussion in other groups
demonstrates, these are only part of the nexus of things, knowledge, rules and
routines that make up the practice of food storage, as highlighted in a second group
discussion, this time in Norfolk:

*R: Bearing in mind that people round our age remember war time and the food we had, the
rations, you made good everything that you could get, nothing was thrown away*
A: We didn't know how old it was did we?
P: Well no, because you went every day to the shop
(Group A)

Although R's discussion of waste echoes that in group E, important distinctions
are introduced by other participants. They suggest that the important changes in
food storage are those related to the knowledge available to consumers, and in the
changing routines of food shopping. Initially, the group move away from this point,
continuing a discussion of wartime rationing that closely parallels that introduced
above. Shortly afterwards however, another participant returns to the question of
changing shopping routines and their relationship with food storage practices:

*J: I think that P made a point about the different way we buy when you said you bought
every day or something which is what you did then, you did more bit shopping rather than
going for a week or a month's shopping so what's in your cupboard is a whole different ball
game anyway isn't it? And we didn't have a fridge, I remember the meat, the larders with
the white netting . . . So you didn't have to look at the sell by date because you bought it that
couple of days and you ate it*
(Group A)

Participants situate their unwillingness to waste food and experiences of wartime
rationing within the shopping routines and food technologies of their early lives.
During the life-time of participants, each of these has changed significantly, with
technological changes in food storage such as the introduction of refrigerators and
freezers (see, e.g. Shove and Southerton 2000), and changes in shopping frequency,
methods and geographies. Older people in the focus groups describe how food
shopping has changed from an everyday activity associated with larders and short
storage times to a weekly or even monthly event linked to cupboards, fridges and
freezers:

J: Every day, we used to go out every day because there were no freezers
K: We don't have a freezer and we shop day to day
*J: My daughters, when they're working, just go shopping and they get for week so that they
haven't got to keep rushing backwards and. . . you know for odds and ends but not for,
I mean they'll know, especially one knows as she writes a list, they're having that Monday,
Tuesday, Wednesday and she writes all down what they're having each day and as I say it's
all in freezer most of the stuff*
(Group B)

The type of food storage technology available is associated with the provisioning
strategy. Freezers and fridges enabled food to be stored safely and kept 'fresh' for
longer, in turn allowing shopping to become less frequent, while a lack of a freezer

is linked with day to day shopping, as suggested by K. It is difficult to determine in which direction this relationship operates, but it is likely that those people who shop more frequently are less likely to have felt the need to purchase a freezer, and this has in turn reinforced this shopping pattern. In these discussions, food storage practices are established through the relations between dispositions, the domestic environment and the technologies within it.

Changing retail movements and environments

The relationship between food storage, technology and shopping routines introduced by discussion of fridge and freezers can be developed by considering changing shopping mobilities. As the following section considers, the changing geographies and mobilities associated with food shopping are important in understanding the context of food storage and its potential contribution to food safety and risk.

Older people, particular those in poor health, on low incomes and in rural areas report difficulty getting to the shops and shopping (McKie 1999, Lumbers and Raats 2006) that are exacerbated by changes in the food retail environment. Foremost among these are the redistribution of food retail and changes in older consumer's ability to access it:

> RM: We've talked about quite a lot of places where you get your food from, whether it gets delivered or things like that, has that changed?
> All: Yes
> D: It used to be the little corner shop
> A: You used to go out with the pram and just go to the corner shop, you don't do that now. I go on a shoppers' bus so I'm a bit limited where I can go anyway
> RM: Is it that the corner shop isn't there?
> A: The corner shop's not there, it used to be just opposite
> (Group E)

For older consumers without access to independent forms of transport, changes in the retail environment are significant. As described earlier, those without cars are able to shop less frequently, prompting changes in diet or planned ventures further afield (Caraher et al. 1998, Coveney and O'Dwyer 2009, Dean et al. 2009). The increasing level of food supply/planning involved in food purchase reflects efforts to maintain and reproduce existing consumption patterns and maintain independence (cf. Lumber and Raats 2006). Hence, older people keep a larger supply of food in the home (Johnson et al. 1998, Turrini et al. 2010), and as focus group participants describe, change their purchasing routines to reflect the exigencies of provisioning and storage:

> JP: We buy Cravendale milk because that lasts a bit longer and we're limited where we can go because we haven't got transport so we would like to go to a farm shop to get things, certain things but it's impossible so we have to make do with Sainsbury's, sometimes we can get to Tesco's if somebody takes us but other than that we can't get to any of these farm shops
> (Group A)

As they do not have access to a car, JP and her husband rely on the smaller Sainsbury's Local convenience store near to their house. Trips to the large Tesco's on the edge of town are impractical without the help of others. They cope by purchasing accordingly, sustaining existing practices by changing the materials that compose them to accommodate changes in mobility. However, when ill or injured, coping mechanisms may be insufficient to maintain practices. Changes in the diet, in shopping routines and in food storage may be enforced, as described below:

> C: I freeze things, I buy things from the butchers, I buy a kilo of chicken fillets and I put two in each, in a bag which is usually about six and I eat two and I put the rest in the freezer. I use the freezer a lot, always for meat, I've always got some frozen vegetables in case I need them but I've got fresh as well, and I use it for bread. If you can't do your shopping, I mean Ted can do some of it but I don't like him doing too much because of his heart and you've always got something in then if you can't get to the shops or the homecare workers don't come. I'm worse now than I used to be at hoarding food because it's become a real issue, if you can't get food, it's very difficult
> M: Absolutely
> C: It must be difficult with a condition like yours to actually have, worry about having enough to eat sometimes
> M: And when you live on your own as well you've got to be sure that you can survive
> C: It seems so remote, it seems such a long distance away, but when John had his heart attack, the home-care started coming and I actually realised that my back was so bad that I can't get to the shop, I can't do my shopping, so they gave me some homecare services but prior to that because he'd been fit and well we'd have done it together and that means him humping ten bags of shopping around and me not carrying anything which is...you see life changes doesn't it, sometimes rather rapidly and rather for the worse sometimes. But I do freeze a lot more now than I used to, it's very useful and then I take things out and put frozen things into the slow cooker and leave it all day, it's very convenient because it's an idle way of cooking I suppose.
> M: Got it sorted ain't she
> C: I had to get it sorted otherwise I wouldn't have had anything to eat
> (Group F)

Changing food storage and provisioning practices are brought about by significant life changes, such as the back injury and a heart attack described by C and a colon operation earlier described by M. It is at this point that the relations between the heterogeneous components of 'safe' everyday consumption become unsustainable and vulnerability slips into risk as the configuration of food practices is changed. New technologies are adopted and the use of existing ones expanded, such as the freezer or the slow cooker, new forms of provisioning are introduced, involving new actors and mobilities, and coping mechanisms such as 'hoarding' emerge that contrast with the everyday shopping described earlier. These changes enable consumers to continue to eat and 'survive', but represent an irreversible shift in the long-reproduced practices associated with safe consumption.

Discussion and conclusions

A number of changes and challenges associated with food and ageing have been identified in existing research. However, no links have been made between these challenges and vulnerability to food-borne illness. The discussions presented in this article suggest that in the case of pathogens such as *L. monocytogenes* which are associated with domestic food storage, much of this study is of relevance. Changes related to older people's mobilities and retail environments represent longer term trends than the recent rise in listeriosis, and are not an explanation for it. Nevertheless, the prevalence of infection among those living in deprived areas and among the elderly (Gillespie *et al.* 2010a, b) suggests that these may represent important and under-examined contributors to food safety risk.

A social practice-based approach to food safety demonstrates the dynamic and fragile nature of practices in the face of social, technological and geographical challenges. It draws attention to the ongoing work that goes into maintaining food 'strategies' through the constant alignment of nexuses of things, knowledge, rules and routines. Further research into the social, economic and geographical contexts of food safety would contribute to opening up distinctions between those who are merely vulnerable to listeriosis and those who become 'at risk'. This may also involve the development and reanalysis of existing datasets. For example, the Nottingham study of Food in Later Life conducted in the mid-1990s (Johnson *et al.* 1998) provides a comprehensive and available dataset related to older people's food practices that could potentially provide a baseline for the new quantitative research suggested by the SSRC (2009).

In addition, focussing on food safety as socially embedded opens the doors to new forms of interventions. At the moment, this is under-recognised in food safety policies that either problematise the behaviour of vulnerable individuals and emphasise their responsibility or that infantilise them and remove responsibility entirely (cf. Hockey and James 1993). Policy interventions that enable consumers to remain independent and that support established food practices – for example by ensuring access to good food delivery services – can make a valuable contribution. In such cases, food safety policy works with, rather than on, consumers.

Note

1. Two groups also included participants younger than 60 who were related to other older group members. It is also important to note here the distinction between different measures of age and ageing. The 'chronological age' of individuals may not equate to other biological, psychological or social measures of ageing (Hockey and James 1993). On these measures, people's age may differ from that of other members of the same cohort. Moreover, the over-60s, as 'older people' are defined by the ACMSF (2009) report, is a diverse group, including at least two generations and individuals at various stages of life and health (SSRC 2009).

References

ACMSF, 2009. *Report on the increased incidence of listeriosis in the UK*. London: Ad Hoc Group on Vulnerable Groups, Advisory Committee on the Microbiological Safety of Food.

Banister, D. and Bowling, A., 2004. Quality of life for the elderly: the transport dimension. *Transport Policy*, 11, 105–115.

Barnes, M., *et al.*, 2006. *The social exclusion of older people: evidence from the first wave of the English longitudinal study of ageing*. London: Office of the Deputy Prime Minister.

Brennan, M., McCarthy, M., and Ritson, C., 2007. Why do consumers deviate from best microbiological food safety advice? An examination of 'high-risk' consumers on the island of Ireland. *Appetite*, 49 (2), 405–418.

Bromley, R.D.F. and Thomas, C.J., 1993. The retail revolution, the carless shopper and disadvantage. *Transactions of the Institute of British Geographers*, 18 (2), 222–236.

Cabinet Office, 2008. *Food: an analysis of the issues*. Discussion Paper. London: Strategy Unit, Cabinet Office.

Caraher, M., *et al.*, 1998. Access to healthy foods: Part I. Barriers to accessing healthy foods: differentials by gender, social class, income and mode of transport. *Health Education Journal*, 57 (3), 191–201.

Cates, S.C., *et al.*, 2006. Older adults' knowledge, attitudes, and practices regarding listeriosis prevention. *Food Protection Trends*, 26 (11), 774–785.

Coveney, J. and O'Dwyer, L., 2009. Effects of mobility and location on food access. *Health and Place*, 15 (1), 45–55.

Cummins, S. and McIntyre, S., 2002. "Food deserts"—evidence and assumption in health policy making. *British Medical Journal*, 325 (7361), 436–438.

Dean, M., *et al.*, 2009. Factors influencing eating a varied diet in old age. *Public Health Nutrition*, 12 (12), 2421–2427.

Evans, D., in press. Beyond the throwaway society: ordinary domestic practice and a sociological approach to household food waste. *Sociology*.

Everts, J. and Jackson, P., 2009. Modernisation and the practices of contemporary food shopping. *Environment and Planning D: Society and Space*, 27 (5), 917–935.

Giles, E., 2009. *Older people and food: a synthesis of evidence.* London: FSA Social Science Research Unit.

Gillespie, I.A., *et al.*, 2010a. Listeria monocytogenes infection in the over-60s in England between 2005 and 2008: a retrospective case-control study utilizing market research panel data. *Foodborne Pathogens and Disease*, 7 (11), 1373–1379.

Gillespie, I.A., *et al.*, 2010b. Human listeriosis in England, 2001–2007: association with neighbourhood deprivation. *Euro Surveillance*, 15 (27), pii=19609.

Goulet, V., *et al.*, 2008. Increasing incidence of listeriosis in France and other European countries. *Emerging Infectious Diseases*, 14 (5), 734–740.

Green, J.M., *et al.*, 2005. Public understanding of food risks in four European countries: a qualitative study. *European Journal of Public Health*, 15 (5), 523–527.

Halkier, B. and Jensen, I., 2011. Methodological challenges in using practice theory in consumption research. Examples from a study on handling nutritional contestations of food consumption. *Journal of Consumer Culture*, 11 (1), 101–123.

Herne, S., 1995. Research on food choice and nutritional status in elderly people: a review. *British Food Journal*, 97 (9), 12–29.

Hockey, J. and James, A., 1993. *Growing up and growing old: ageing and dependency in the life course.* London: Sage Publications.

Hutton, D., 2009. *Look out for listeria: reducing food poisoning in the over 60s.* Speech by Deirdre Hutton, Chair, at Food Standards Agency Parliamentary reception, Members' Dining Room, Palace of Westminster, Wednesday, 17 June 2009.

Jackson, P., *et al.*, 2006. Retail restructuring and consumer choice 2. Understanding consumer choice at the household level. *Environment and Planning A*, 38 (1), 47–67.

Jackson, P. and Holbrook, B., 1995. Multiple meanings: shopping and the cultural politics of identity. *Environment and Planning A*, 27 (12), 1913–1930.

Johnson, A.E., *et al.*, 1998. Food safety knowledge and practice among elderly people living at home. *Journal of Epidemiology and Community Health*, 52 (11), 745–748.

Kitzinger, J., 1995. Qualitative research: introducing focus groups. *British Medical Journal*, 311 (7000), 299–302.

Kitzinger, J. and Barbour, R., 1999. *Developing focus group research: politics, theory and practice.* London: Sage Publications.

Lumbers, M. and Raats, M.M., 2006. Food choices in later life. *In*: R. Shepherd and M. Raats, eds. *Psychology of food choice.* Wallingford, UK: CABI Pub in association with the Nutrition Society, Frontiers in Nutritional Science, no 3.

Maycroft, N., 2009. Not moving things along: hoarding, clutter and other ambiguous matter. *Journal of Consumer Behaviour*, 8 (6), 354–364.

McKie, L., 1999. Older people and food: independence, locality and diet. *British Food Journal*, 101 (7), 528–536.

Meah, A. and Watson, M., 2011. Saints and slackers: challenging discourses about the decline of domestic cooking. *Sociological Research* [online], 16 (2), 6. Available from: http://www.socresonline.org.uk/16/2/6.html

Milton, A. and Mullan, B., 2010. Consumer food safety education for the domestic environment: a systematic review. *British Food Journal*, 112 (9), 1003–1022, Emerald Group.

Reckwitz, A., 2002. Toward a theory of social practices: a development in culturalist theorizing. *European Journal of Social Theory*, 5 (2), 243–263.

Shove, E. and Pantzar, M., 2010. Understanding innovation in practice: a discussion of the production and re-production of Nordic walking. *Technology Analysis and Strategic Management*, 22 (4), 447–461.

Shove, E. and Southerton, D., 2000. Defrosting the freezer: from novelty to convenience: a narrative of normalization. *Journal of Material Culture*, 5 (3), 301–319.

SSRC, 2009. *L. monocytogenes and food storage and food handling practices of the over 60s at home*. Report of the Social Science Research Committee Working Group on Listeria.

Terpstra, M.J., *et al.*, 2005. Food storage and disposal: consumer practices and knowledge. *British Food Journal*, 107 (7), 526–533.

Turrini, A., *et al.*, 2010. The informal networks in food procurement by older people—a cross European comparison. *Ageing International*, 35 (4), 253–275.

Warde, A., 2005. Consumption and theories of practice. *Journal of Consumer Culture*, 5 (2), 131–153.

Wilson, L.C., Alexander, A., and Lumbers, M., 2004. Food access and dietary variety among older people. *International Journal of Retail & Distribution Management*, 32 (2), 109–22.

WRAP, 2008. *The food we waste*. Banbury: Waste and Resources Action Programme.

Wrigley, N., 2002. "Food deserts" in British cities: policy context and research priorities. *Urban Studies*, 39 (11), 2029–2040.

Preventing anxiety: a qualitative study of fish consumption and pregnancy

Helene Brembeck

Centre for Consumer Science, University of Gothenburg, 405 30 Gothenburg, Sweden

Starting from theories of anxiety as social practice, this article explores the contested landscape of health, risks associated with fish consumption and pregnancy in Sweden, and the way risk communicators and pregnant women navigate this landscape. This article argues that the risk analysis by the Swedish National Food Administration is a good example of the practices of definition and annihilation of subjects and objects of anxiety. It shows that the creation of anxious subjects is counteracted by two means in the brochures and on the website of the National Food Administration (NFA): by placing information about pregnancy and fish within a risk discourse, and by liberal governance. This article concludes that, although pregnant women manage and control anxiety during pregnancy by several practices, this strategy by the NFA does not make them feel safe and secure, which is the basic duty of the NFA, but rather bolsters their feeling that you cannot ever feel safe, you always have to anticipate that something bad might happen.

Introduction

Sweden has a long tradition of fish consumption. Fish is perceived as a healthy and necessary part of the diet, not least by authorities such as the National Food Administration (NFA). Today, the NFA recommends two to three servings of fish a week for all Swedes. In recent years, the healthiness of fish has, however, been seriously contested. For more than 30 years, fish has been increasingly drawn into discourses of risk and anxiety, as various health dangers have been detected. The most notable risks involve pesticide residuals and *Listeria* in fish. Fish consumption now resides in a misty domain of health, risk, and the sciences of toxicology and nutrition (Ådnegård Skarstad 2008). This is particularly true for pregnant women, who have increasingly been identified as the main risk group by the NFA.

Starting from theories of anxiety as social practice (Jackson and Everts 2010), this article explores the contested landscape of health, risks associated with fish consumption and pregnancy, and the way risk communicators and pregnant women navigate this landscape. The study is part of the ERC-funded program *Consumer Culture in an Age of Anxiety* (CONANX), which focuses on anxiety at the intersection of markets and morality, trust, risk and health, where one of the work packages is specifically devoted to consumer understandings of risk, anxiety and trust (http://www.sheffield.ac.uk/conanx/index.html). Research that forms the background to the program has shown that fear is 'a social or collective experience rather than an individual state,' and that fear is 'embedded in a network of moral and political geographies' (Pain and Smith 2008). Furthermore, sites of social anxiety are converging with discourses of risk, frequently containing a strongly moral dimension which Hier (2003) describes in terms of the 'moralization of risk.' Hier identifies a growing tension between the 'techno-scientific rationalities' of expert systems and what he calls the 'social rationalities' of everyday living. The gap between these different rationalities is a fertile ground for the development of social anxiety, as this and other studies from the CONANX program show (Milne 2011).

In this article, I will give a brief overview of risk communication about fish to pregnant women in Sweden, and discuss the risk management and risk communication practices of the NFA. I will then go on to discuss women's strategies and anxieties about fish during pregnancy from a perspective that focuses on everyday practices and attunement. I use theories on the modulation of affect that have been developed in the program to discuss the difficulties of risk communication and the unpredictability of the consumers' responses (Milne *et al.* 2011).

Anxiety as social practice

Jackson and Everts (2010) explore anxiety as a social practice that consists of a combination of affective experiences, bodily reactions and behavioral responses (Wilkinson 2001). They argue that anxieties emerge through an 'event' that disrupts everyday life by forcing a realization of mortality or meaninglessness. It is through the event that the 'wholesome experience of one's being-in-the-world collapses into subjects and objects of anxiety' (Jackson and Everts 2010, p. 2798). The disintegration of everyday life leads to the adoption of a set of practices in order to manage the anxiety. The first of these is the practice of framing, or defining, the event that produces anxiety. Here scientific or expert practices are of particular importance. Consumers also engage in various practices to keep themselves informed, and to understand what is going on. The second practice is that of annihilation, which includes all the actions and statements that are specifically designed or employed to destroy the objects and subjects of anxiety. If annihilation of the object is not possible or only partially successful, such as is the case of pesticides or listeria in fish, a third practice is employed, based upon the constant effort that is required to retrieve people from their anxious subject positions. In this case, the creation of anxious subjects must be constantly combated.

Jackson and Everts (2010) contend that any kind of social anxiety can be understood more thoroughly by focusing on these interweaving sets of practices. To understand the outcomes of a given social anxiety, we need to examine how the whole flow of everyday life becomes reworked in the face of the disruptive state of anxiety, and we need to understand how they are articulated within different 'communities of practice,' from the way in which government institutions are organized to identify and handle possible outbreaks of anxiety to the way in which our everyday practices of shopping, cooking and eating are affected.

Materials and methods

This article draws on a study conducted during 2010 which used several materials and methods. For an historic overview, all editions of information manuals on dietary advice about fish produced by the NFA from 1968 up to 2009 were studied, a total of eight editions. Texts, pictures, and communication strategies in the brochures were scrutinized and compared. To get an overview of the process of risk analysis by the NFA, a group of officials who are responsible for the risk analysis process were interviewed. I spent 1 day visiting the agency in Uppsala, where I conducted a 2 h interview with the group of four persons, and a shorter separate interview with the person responsible for risk communication. I was also given names of senior employees who could tell me more about the NFA's former work with fish. I took the opportunity to e-mail some more questions after my visit, and was given prompt and informative answers.

This article also draws on a number of interviews with a group of nine women with small babies. In Sweden, all parents are invited to attend parents' group meetings at maternity care centers during their pregnancy and the first months after the delivery. I was allowed access to one of these groups, and the women agreed to meet with me specifically to discuss the issues I was interested in. I arranged a first group discussion at the maternity care center, when the babies were 5 months old, which focussed on the issue of information about fish during pregnancy. During the following months, I conducted five individual follow-up interviews and took part in three group discussions on this issue. The interviews and discussions were done at the homes of one of them, or on one occasion during a picnic in a park. They were tape recorded and transcribed and resulted in a little over 100 pages of written text.

The women were all first-time mothers, aged 25–34 and lived in a central part of Gothenburg. They had not known each other prior to their pregnancy, but had been part of the same parents' group at their local maternity care center, since their births were planned for the same month (January 2010). They continued to meet every Tuesday during the first year of the parental leave (which is 18 months in Sweden, the mother usually takes her leave during the first year). They had urban lifestyles, liked to stroll around the city streets and parks with their babies, socializing with friends, shopping, having a cup of coffee together, etc. They were socio-economically diverse. There were service workers (such as a shop assistant), professionals (such as a nurse), and academics (such as a bio-technician working at an advanced level in a major pharmaceutical company).

I conducted interviews with two of the midwives at the maternity care center that the women attended, and who had conveyed the information and brochures to them. I also studied the discussion forum on the NFA website and its information site on Facebook aimed at pregnant women, and the questions and answers posted there. Finally, I contacted representatives of the Maternal and Child Health Psychologists' Association. Their members support local midwives in their contacts with pregnant women, and they have considerable expertise in women's worries during pregnancy throughout Sweden.

Anxiety prevention

The practices of risk analysis by the NFA are a good example of the practices of definition and annihilation of subjects and objects of anxiety proposed by Jackson and Everts. Risk analysis is about making dangers manageable by turning them into risks. It is about preventing anxiety in a sensible way, without frightening consumers. This is the mission of the NFA, I was told, and this is the daily task of about 300 persons working in the three separate departments of risk evaluation, risk handling and risk communication.

At the start there is no risk, just a possible danger, and the duty of the risk evaluators is to assess whether the danger is a risk, and thus can be passed on along the risk analysis chain. Risk evaluation is described as a strictly scientific process. It is about 'weighing the danger (of a substance) against the likelihood that something will happen and how many might be affected,' according to the officials. There are 'tolerable intakes,' and security factors, the amounts of for example dioxins in fish must be 100 times less than what has been proven harmful in animal studies. If the risk evaluators conclude that a large fraction of the population will consume an unacceptable amount of the food, danger has turned into a risk and the case is passed on to the risk handlers.

The risk handlers consider other things than pure scientific facts. They have to weigh risks versus public anxiety (and maybe other aspects such as the possibility of banning a product). Often there is not a great risk but a great concern among consumers, and then the risk handlers decide that the NFA needs to improve communication about the case with consumers. The case is passed to the risk communication department.

The risk communicators have used essentially the same strategy to inform expectant mothers about risks for many years: divide fish in three categories, namely fish you can eat as often as you like, fish you should eat only now and then, and fish you should avoid altogether. The species in the three categories remain the same over time. From this point of view, it is easy to do the right thing. In recent years, the brochures have been supplemented by a Facebook site and a pocket guide that can be downloaded and printed from the website. The latest innovation is a system in which it is possible to send text messages from a cell phone, and receive answers from officials at the NFA right away. The information is consistent, independent of the communication channel used.

The NFA is a well-functioning machine for anxiety prevention. Framing dangers as risks that can be calculated, and thus managed, is the NFA's way of preventing anxieties becoming uncontrollable and giving rise to panic. It is also its way of eliminating responsibility. If the officials perform their duties of risk analysis correctly, they have no responsibility if something goes wrong and unwanted effects occur. The staff can handle all known risks, they argue.

Obviously, risk analysis is not a neutral instrument. As Ådnegård Skarstad (2008) shows in her Norwegian study of fish and health, practices of risk assessment contribute to shaping the definition of fish as food in a specific way: as an issue of risk or non-risk, which in turn makes it difficult to establish fish as healthy. This suggests that rather than being a neutral tool, risk assessment is a technology with the potential of transforming the cultural position of fish.

Fighting the anxious subject

As stated above, if annihilation of the object is not possible or only partially possible, constant effort is required to counteract the creation of anxious subjects. In the brochures and on the website of the NFA this is done by two means: by placing information about pregnancy and fish within a risk discourse, and by liberal governance.

Only one substance is mentioned in the 1971 brochure, mercury, and fishermen and anglers are highlighted as the main risk groups. We learn from the 1992 edition that a very small amount of mercury can harm the nervous system of the fetus, and the risk scenario is broadened to include another five harmful substances, including caesium. Listeria is introduced in the 2003 brochure, and expectant mothers are now warned of eating marinated and smoked fish, and sushi that has not been freshly prepared and recently wrapped. Listeria can harm the fetus and cause miscarriage, we learn. Not only water and fish may be dangerous, but also packaging. The 2009 brochure includes a further range of harmful substances in other kinds of food, such as caffeine, vitamin A (in liver), vitamin pills, ginseng and other health food products and, of course, alcohol.

Coupled with a changing riskscape, the increasing fusion of health and risk information, and toxicological and nutritional facts, pointed to by Ådnegård Skarstad (2008), is obvious. You must not only avoid harmful substances: you must ensure that you consume a whole range of healthy substances: vitamin D and omega-3 from fish (omega-3 is mentioned for the first time in the 2003 edition), and folic acid, iodine and iron from other foods. A landscape of good and bad substances opens up.

This is consistent with Ruhl's Canadian study of information manuals given to pregnant women (Ruhl 1999). There is now no 'no risk' category in these manuals, she argues. Threat is everywhere; no one is entirely safe, merely more or less statistically vulnerable. Ruhl concludes that more than anything else the 'risk society' exists in perpetual anxiety, because the things most feared (pollution, toxic side effects, miscarriage, deformed babies) are only visible when their effects are manifested. This climate of fear and anxiety exists in a complex dialectic with science, being both fuelled by and allayed by science. This dichotomy arises because it is scientific progress that results in the potential for identifying risk factors and thus proliferating 'risky' situations – and the advancement of prenatal diagnostic techniques, for instance which illuminate a whole new set of 'risk factors' (Ruhl 1999, p. 102).

In the realm of pregnancy, the risks that are the subject of social commentary are almost exclusively risks to the fetus. This is reminiscent of what Ruddick (1994) refers to as 'natal thinking.' Natal thinking is a state of 'active waiting' in which the relationship between the woman and fetus is characterized by responsibility, care, and dependence. A major shift in pregnancy discourses in recent years has been the increasing construction of the 'fetal person' (Daniels 1993, Ruddick 2007), which sees the woman herself as little more than a container for the fetus during pregnancy (Young 1990, Bailey 2001). While concern in the past was more focused on maternal health, today it focuses on the health of the unborn child (Brembeck 1992).

None of the NFA brochures, however, present recommendations, prescription or guidelines: they present solely advice. In communicating with consumers, the risk communicators are anxious not to be perceived as guardians, to be controlling, convicting, or as giving lectures or prescriptions. Their ambition is not to tell women what to do and what not to do. Instead, they want the NFA to be a reliable but friendly partner, giving consumers good advice that they can follow if they want to. It must be the consumers' choice. They do not want to be accused of playing the role of 'nanny state.' They are working in the best interests of the consumers, but are not being bossy and intruding into their lives. They want to behave like modern parents: sensitive to their children's needs, but always letting them have the last say. On the other hand, consumers are perceived as somewhat wilful and errant children. You never really know how to approach them or how they will react to your advice. All you can do is to be patient and be there if and when they need you.

Ruhl (1999) argues that this model of regulating pregnancy through liberal governance (Rose 1993, Valverde 1996) that is currently dominant mobilizes a discourse of risk, and of risk prevention and reduction that enlists the co-operation of the 'responsible' pregnant woman. Responsibility is equated with the capacity to behave rationally: the term presupposes a calculation of expected benefits and risks, and a decision to follow the path with the greatest possibility of benefit with the least risk. In this sense, a discussion of responsibility within liberal regimes is also a discussion of morality – behaving responsibly is a moral act. As argued by Ruhl (1999, p. 96), risk discourses depend on the entrenchment of a sense of personal responsibility, which is downplayed and may be lost if activities are simply forbidden. Casting the pregnant woman as an agent in her pregnancy is not necessarily a negative development – on the contrary, the 'responsible' pregnant woman also installs women as active participants in their reproductive capacities.

Modulation and affect

From this overview, it is clear that when women become pregnant and receive dietary advice at the maternity care centers, they enter a contested domain. Different discourses are crowding, being delivered in both verbal and written information: about the female responsibility to care for her body and health, and most pertinently for the body and health of the fetus, and a woman's duty to listen to the experts but eventually to guide herself. There are also conflicting discourses about fish as healthy and as harmful, with evidence being presented from toxicology on the one hand and from nutrition on the other.

It is also evident that the information from the NFA involves more than rational statements at a cognitive level. It is not only packed with moral discourses: it is presented with an affective tone. Although the affective nature of food is well established, Milne *et al.* (2011) argue that the importance of affect and emotion in the circulation of information about food remains neglected. Inspired by the 'affective turn' in social sciences, the authors 'consider anxiety as an affect, as a processual transformation of bodily capacity or power to act, conceived as an ability to affect and be affected by others' (2011). Not only the content of information is important, but its affective consequences, its role in *affecting* the reader.

As I will show, information to pregnant women about the risks of consuming hazardous fish is especially pertinent in this respect. These are not just any kind of risks, but risks of exactly the existential character that Jackson and Everts (2010) envision, with the power to force a realization of mortality or meaninglessness, in this case of the danger of lethal harm to your unborn child. The NFA states that the consumption of risky fish during pregnancy belongs to the few certain dangers that must be kept as low as possible; substances that cause interference in the reproductive organs or neurotoxicological effects, and thus endanger the survival of the human species.

Milne *et al.* (2011) suggest, following Massumi (2005), that the movement of concerns, anxieties or worries involves more than a simple linear model of transmission, it is about modulation. In Massumi's (2005) discussion of fear and efforts to communicate the possibility of terrorist attacks in post-9/11 America, he argues that threat alerts performed the role of affective 'modulation,' by which the majority of the US population was brought into a state of continual, but 'appropriate' anxiety or fear.

.This resonates well with the objective of the NFA to promote the capacities of pregnant women to act rationally in encounters with potentially harmful fish.

Importantly, however, Milne *et al.* (2011) highlight that the consequences of the circulation of affect are unpredictable. As Massumi (2005, p. 34) suggests, in the case of terror alerts:

> ...the social environment within which government now operated was of such complexity that it made a mirage of any idea that there could be a one-to-one correlation between official speech or image production and the form and content of response.

Summing up, Milne *et al.* (2011) suggest that the concept of 'modulation' represents a more accurate description of the circulation of affect through multiple media (or 'milieux'), one that captures fluctuations in affect while remaining sensitive to the unpredictable and uncertain products of affective encounters.

Localizing anxiety

> Hello! I was at a spa last weekend and had forgotten the booklet on dietary guidelines for pregnant women at home. I had previously notified the restaurant that I am pregnant. When I looked at the menu there was walleye. I said that I did not think I could eat it. The waiter, however, was confident that walleye from Lake Hjälmaren (close to Stockholm in the eastern part of Sweden) was OK to eat if you are pregnant, that there is no danger at all. He also said that the fish was farmed...
> So I ate the fish. When I got home, I saw in the booklet that you should eat walleye a maximum of 2-3 times per year. I would not eat anything that is bad for my baby and felt a bit cheated by the restaurant. I have searched online and found some evidence to suggest that fish from Lake Hjälmaren does not contain as much toxic residue, do you know anything about this? My question is, do you know if it is better to eat fish from Lake Hjälmaren than other freshwater fish, from the point of view of pollution and pesticide residue?

The questioner is a 28-year-old woman who is 5 months pregnant, and the question is one of many similar at NFA's Facebook site.

The answer is brief and reassuring:

> Hello! You need not worry! The fish you ate was farmed, and farmed fish have much lower levels because the feed is 'clean' and controlled.

Women are aware that the everyday practices of shopping for food, cooking, and eating need to be reconsidered when they become pregnant to protect the fetus from harmful substances. The nine women interviewed during this study reported that the first thing they did when they found out that they were pregnant, and even at the stage of planning to conceive, was an intense activity of 'framing,' of searching for information about diet and risks and how to behave. They had all received the brochures about fish consumption from the maternity care center during their pregnancy. They all knew about the NFA. Several of them had looked for information about fish at the NFA website, and they trusted without reservation the information they found there. They consider it to be the best and most up-to-date information available. This agrees with the results of surveys carried out by the NFA, stating that 87% of pregnant women are aware of the advice given and brochures published by the NFA.

This also highlights a new space in which the politics of pregnancy is played out in the twenty-first century, through the virtual community of internet chat rooms and health sites (Fox *et al.* 2009, pp. 67–68). The interviewed women talked in very appreciative terms about the possibility to pose questions on Facebook, and they were lyrical about the new opportunity to ask questions by SMS, which was introduced just before Christmas 2010. 'It is fantastic' one of them exclaimed, 'that you are able to send a query when you are sitting in a restaurant and get an answer immediately.'

It is evident that the NFA advice exists within an ecology of information sources including the media, friends, family, and other sources. Sometimes you also get more or less unwanted 'good advice' from complete strangers. As pregnant you become a public person and open to public scrutiny. As one of the respondents in Fox *et al.* (2007, p. 64) study states: 'We've all had experiences where complete strangers told us what to do, or what not to do.' Scientific 'knowledge' regarding pregnancy is readily available to anybody who wishes to hear it and over time certain discourses (such as the harmful effects of smoking and drinking) become naturalized and seen as 'common sense.' Such public 'knowledge' is used to construct people in their role as societal supervisors of women's behavior, and anyone who chooses to deviate from these norms opens themselves up to potential criticisms of their irresponsibility towards the 'fetal person' (Fox *et al.* 2007).

The cumulative result of the wanted and unwanted advice is often overwhelming to pregnant women (Ruhl 1999). Also in their British study, Fox *et al.* (2007, p. 67) show how freedom of access to information leads many women to feel that there is almost an overavailability of information, making it difficult to decipher what the real 'risks' are. Also, in spite of the possibility of instant advice by the use of SMS, much of the discussion in the Gothenburg women's group resembles the question posed at the NFA's Facebook site quoted above. Here is an excerpt from a discussion of listeria in marinated fish.

> Interviewer: It (Listeria) can also be found in marinated fish...
> Kajsa: Yes, I didn't eat marinated salmon.
> Agnes: No, it was the only thing I didn't...
> Linda: Cold-smoked...
> Kajsa: Not warm-smoked either. But I did actually. Because I didn't know...
> Karin: I didn't know
> Agneta: I didn't know either
> Eva: No....
> Karin: I thought you could eat warm-smoked...
> Kajsa: No, apparently not.
> Klara: Yes, you can eat warm-smoked...though I don't think...
> Anna: Yes, warm-smoked salmon is OK...but herring
> Linda: Yes, it is probably true.
> Klara: Yes, you can eat warm-smoked herring.
> Karin: I am sure you are right.

Obviously, the NFA's communication does not always generate the desired affective responses. Anxieties are not only, or not primarily, rational, cognitive or psychological: they are, as Jackson and Everts (2010, pp. 22–23) state, social, practical and practiced. It is this sense of tacit understanding that anxiety threatens to undermine when people feel unable to deal with the threatening situations in which they find themselves.

Navigating the riskscape

Pregnancy is a biological process, but exists within the social, economic, political, and cultural realms. It is, furthermore, both spatially and temporally limited (Longhurst 1999, p. 89). Women in different places experience pregnancy in a variety of different ways. Individuals may ignore experts and decide for themselves what constitutes healthy and moral self-management (Lindsay 2010, p. 484). Others may seek to balance and combine contradictory imperatives in their everyday consumption practices. It has also been shown that the extent to which women follow or reject advice depends upon several factors including age, education, social class, and the number of previous pregnancies. Women are much more relaxed about following 'rules' and more liable to trust their 'embodied knowledge' during their second pregnancy (Fox *et al.*, p. 67).

In their study of the production of 'authoritative knowledge' in American pre-natal care, Markens *et al.* (1997) argue that women often balance adjustments in their diets to provide acceptable solutions for both themselves and their unborn child. Also the women of this study revealed themselves as active consumers of advice, picking and choosing which bits to follow and actively seeking advice via internet sites, books and magazines. As in other studies of risk perception and risk handling by consumers, these women develop practices to handle the situation and to eliminate the anxiety-producing objects as far as possible. The practices developed include the use of rules of thumb. The most obvious is that since these women are living on the Swedish west coast – and not by the Baltic Sea or close to any lakes – they exempt themselves from the risk group with respect to pollutants and pesticide residuals. They are not at risk since they only eat fish from the clean waters off the west coast. They do not have to worry.

They concentrate instead on Listeria in, for example, sushi and smoked salmon, which are part of their everyday food practices. But although some have been anxious, and some not, none of them have been really afraid of Listeria and they think they have been muddling through their consumption in an 'OK' way. The women are well attuned to the communications on listeriosis, which they consider a potential risk in their everyday life. Although this is something they keep in mind more or less all the time, they are not necessarily anxious, but rather are enabled to act. Most develop coping strategies that enable them to avoid anxious encounters and feel safe, even to the extent that some Gothenburg sushi restaurants have started serving *mamma sushi* (Mummy sushi), which is sushi that is based on avocado, crabfish, shrimp and omelet instead of raw fish, in order to keep their young female customers.

When attunement is not enough

While the risk of listeriosis is a more or less everyday concern for the 'sushi-generation,' the young mothers interviewed were not well attuned to other anxieties, such as pesticide residues, in regard to fish and pregnancy. For these young women living by the 'clean waters' of the Swedish west coast, pesticides are not a great worry. Their level of affective attunement is low, such that anxiety emerges in sudden encounters.

In group discussions, some of the women described the bodily activation caused by eating fish from the blacklist, such as Atlantic halibut or Baltic herring. They describe the bodily reaction that came before the intellectual realization of what they had done, displaying vivid gestures of disgust, as if they try to vomit the food out of their bodies. They depicted the panic and showed with facial expressions and body language how they became petrified with fear, calming down only after reasoning with themselves over the actual risk:

> Kajsa: I panicked, I was at a wedding and we had Atlantic halibut and obviously you should not eat Atlantic halibut I had heard from somewhere. I just... Help! [Takes the throat, eyes widened and opens her mouth in horror]... you know afterwards. I had no idea about it.
> Anna: We were in Österlen [in southern Sweden] and then I found that I had eaten Baltic herring two consecutive days. And you should only do that a maximum of twice a year. I realised it afterwards. At first I was terrified.

These quotes describe moments of large and sudden shocks, pre-emptive moments when the possibility of harming an unborn child for life suddenly becomes perceptible. It takes a few moments of pure panic before cognition catches up, the women start reasoning with themselves and the event is orientated, delimited and can be dealt with.

The case of fish consumption among Swedish women again demonstrates the multiple pathways and bodies through which anxiety is produced, notably in the form of encounters with forbidden fish. The world 'collapses into subjects and objects of anxiety' (Jackson and Everts 2010, p. 2798). However, as Milne *et al.* (2011) argue, such events also show the unpredictable nature of institutional interventions into food safety, and the importance of existing bodily activations and social networks in shaping affective responses. Conceived of in terms of anxiety, the production and circulation of anxiety is reliant on the existence of an affective attunement, without which the modulation of affect produces little response.

Conclusions

This study has shown that there is a tension between the expert system of the NFA and the everyday lives of pregnant women in regard to the management of risks concerning fish in pregnancy, and that this tension gives rise to anxiety. The phases of framing, annihilating, and retrieving from anxiety are basically the same, but the logics and contexts are different. The risk analysis of the NFA is a strictly scientific process, and the staff firmly believes that the advice is consistent, transparent and easy to follow. Women's everyday lives are filled with competing discourses about health, food, and pregnancy from experts as well as laypersons, family and friends. It is also evident that the information from the NFA is packed with moral discourses and is presented in a moral tone. The risk analysis of the NFA can be understood in terms of affect modulation, making aware without frightening.

Affect modulation cannot, however, be understood as a linear exercise of power on consumer bodies. The women in this study develop ways of using information to resist authorities and empower themselves, to attune to the information. They use a variety of sources to make decisions about their food and eating practices, and place themselves within various discourses of good motherhood, expert advice, food and health that are both time and space-specific. Only when attunement is not enough, when unexpected things happen, does a sudden panic arise, before the women's cognitive processes catch up and order is restored.

One might conclude that the NFA's ambition to give friendly advice, a few warning signs in terms of lists of fish with different degrees of alarm leaving the interpretation and the decisions to the women, leads to a strategy that does not make them feel safe and secure, which is the basic duty of the NFA. The NFA rather bolsters the women's feeling that you cannot ever feel safe, you always have to anticipate that something bad might happen. Although you can keep anxiety at bay most of the time, it is still somewhere in the back of your head, and pops up as an immediate bodily reaction of total fear the moment you realize that you have eaten a piece of Baltic herring. More and more advanced technologies of modulation are needed to keep anxiety about food and pregnancy at bay and to prevent full panic. The readiness of the NFA to always be there to give a helping hand, including the use of instant interactive means such as Facebook and SMS, is not only a way to fight the anxious subject that agrees with the women's preferences, it is a way of keeping pregnancy and food steadfast within the realm of risk and anxiety.

Acknowledgments

The author would like to thank Peter Jackson, Richard Milne, Jakob Wenzer, and Maria Brodin for discussion and support in the writing of this article. The research discussed here is being undertaken as part of work package four of the CONANX project, funded by the European Research Council (www.sheffield.ac.uk/conanx).

References

Ådnegård Skarstad, G., 2008. Balancing fish: a meeting between food safety and nutrition in an assessment of benefits and risks. *Distinktion. Scandinavian Journal of Social Theory*, 9 (1), 99–114.

Bailey, L., 2001. Gender shows: first-time mothers and embodied selves. *Gender and Society*, 15, 110–129.

Brembeck, H., 1992. *Inte bara mamma: En etnologisk studie av unga kvinnors syn på moderskap, barn och familj*. Göteborg: Etnologiska föreningen i Västsverige.

Daniels, C.R., 1993. *At women's expense: state power and the politics of foetal rights*. Cambridge, MA: Harvard University Press.

Fox, R., Nicholson, P., and Heffernan, K., 2009. Pregnancy police? Maternal bodies, surveillance and food. *In*: P. Jackson, ed. *Changing families, changing food*. Houndmills, Basingstoke: Palgrave Macmillan, 57–74.

Hier, S., 2003. Risk and panic in late modernity: implications of converging sites of social anxiety. *British Journal of Sociology*, 54, 3–20.

Jackson, P. and Everts, J., 2010. Anxiety as social practice. *Environment and Planning A*, 42 (11), 2791–2806.

Lindsay, J., 2010. Healthy living guidelines and the disconnect with everyday life. *Critical Public Health*, 20 (4), 475–487.

Longhurst, R., 1999. Pregnant bodies, public scrutiny: 'giving' advice to pregnant women. *In*: E.K. Teather, ed. *Embodied geographies: spaces, bodies and rites of passage*. London: Routledge, 78–90.

Markens, S., Browner, C., and Press, N., 1997. Feeding the foetus: on interrogating the notion of maternal-foetal conflict. *Feminist Studies*, 23, 351–372.

Massumi, B., 2005. Fear (the spectrum said). *Positions*, 13 (1), 31–48.

Milne, R., 2011. A focus group study of food safety practices in relation to listeriosis among the over-60s. *Critical Public Health*, 21 (4), 485–495.

Milne, R., *et al.*, 2011. Fraught cuisine: food scares and the modulation of anxieties. *Distinktion: Scandinavian Journal of Social Theory*, 12 (2), 177–192.

Pain, R. and Smith, S., 2008. Fear: critical geopolitics and everyday life. *In*: R. Pain and S. Smith, eds. *Fear: critical geopolitics and everyday life*. Aldershot: Ashgate, 1–19.

Rose, N., 1993. Government, authority and expertise in advanced liberalism. *Economy and Society*, 33 (3), 283–300.

Ruddick, S., 1994. Thinking mothers/conceiving birth. *In*: D. Bassin, M. Honey and M. Mahrer Kaplan, eds. *Representations of motherhood*. New Haven, CT and New York, NY: Yale University Press, 29–46.

Ruddick, S., 2007. At the horizons of the subject: neo-liberalism, neo-conservatism and the rights of the child, part one. *Gender, Place and Culture*, 14, 513–526.

Ruhl, L., 1999. Liberal governance and parental care: risk and regulation in pregnancy. *Economy and Society*, 28 (1), 95–117.

Valverde, M., 1996. *The age of light, soap, and water*. Toronto: McClelland & Stewart.

Wilkinson, I., 2001. *Anxiety in a risk society*. London: Routledge.

Young, I.M., 1990. *Throwing like a girl and other essays in feminist psychology and social meaning*. Bloomington, IN: Indiana University Press.

Index